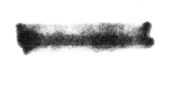

Baby to Parent,
Parent to Baby

Baby to Parent, Parent to Baby

A GUIDE TO DEVELOPING PARENT-CHILD INTERACTION IN THE FIRST TWELVE MONTHS

Ira J. Gordon

DEAN, SCHOOL OF EDUCATION
UNIVERSITY OF NORTH CAROLINA
AT CHAPEL HILL

Illustrated by Ethel Gold

St. Martin's Press
New York

Library of Congress Cataloging in Publication Data

Gordon, Ira J
  Baby to parent, parent to baby.

  1. Parent and child.   2. Infant psychology.
I. Title.

HQ774.G67   649'.122   76-62768
ISBN 0-312-06448-9
ISBN 0-312-06449-7 pbk.

For my wife, Esther, who began my education as a father, who has, through the years, continued to teach me about parenting, exemplifying "loving and learning," who read, corrected, and commented on the manuscript; and for our children, Bonnie and Gary, who also read and commented on portions of this manuscript, who continue to demonstrate curiosity, commitment, and self-reliance. This book, in its germination over two decades ago and in its fruition now, has been truly a family affair.

Acknowledgments

The ideas in *Baby to Parent, Parent to Baby* reflect not only my own work but also that of many other child-development specialists—scientists, pediatricians, and educators. The following list represents only those whose publications, if this were a scholarly book, would have been cited in the usual style, accompanied by bibliographic references. I hope they will accept this means of acknowledgment as an indication of my respect for their work and for their contributions to my thought and practice.

Mary Ainsworth
John A. B. Allan
Tina Appleton
Nancy Bayley
Richard Q. Bell
Sylvia Bell
E. Kuno Beller
Herbert G. Birch
John Bowlby
Yvonne Brackbill
T. Barry Brazelton
Sylvia Brody
Jerome Bruner
Dorothy Burlingham
Justin D. Call
Genevieve Carpenter
Stella Chess
Allison Clarke-Stewart
Rachel Clifton
Herbert J. Cohen
Therese Gouin Decarie
Peggy Emerson
Erik H. Erikson
Sybille Escalona
Daniel G. Freedman
Anna Freud
Arnold Gesell
Susan Goldberg
Murray B. Gordon

Grace Heider
J. McVicker Hunt
Dorothy Huntington
Frances L. Ilg
Jerome Kagan
John Kennell
Marshall Klaus
Anneliese F. Korner
J. Ronald Lally
Michael Lewis
Eleanor Maccoby
Myrtle McGraw
George H. Mead
Esther Milner
Roeanne P. Moreno
Howard Moss
Gardner Murphy
Lois B. Murphy
Katherine Nelson
Ronald K. Parker
David R. Pederson
Jean Piaget
Emmi Pikler
Daniel A. Prescott
Sally Provence
M.P.M. Richards
James Robertson
Joyce Robertson
Mary Budd Rowe

H. Rudolph Schaffer
Gerald Stechler
Lawrence Taft
Evelyn B. Thoman
A. Thomas
Ina Uzgiris
Mary F. Waldrop
John S. Watson
George M. Weller
Peter Wolff
Leon J. Yarrow
Robert W. Zaslow

I am especially indebted to Tina Appleton, Mary Ainsworth, A. Thomas and Herbert G. Birch, John Bowlby, Jerome Bruner, Stella Chess, Rachel Clifton, Erik H. Erikson, Sybille Escalona, Susan Goldberg, Lois B. and Gardner Murphy, Jean Piaget, Evelyn Thoman; to E. Kuno Beller, J. Ronald Lally, Roeanne P. Moreno, and Leon J. Yarrow, my colleagues in the Social Emotional project sponsored by the Office of Child Development, United States Department of Health, Education, and Welfare, and the University of Florida College of Education; to Barry Guinagh and Robert Jester, my co-workers in the various infant projects of the Institute for the Development of Human Resources at the College of Education, University of Florida; and to the families, paraprofessionals and graduate students with whom we worked.

The materials in the section "Difficult Baby" in the chapter on the second and third months are extensively adapted from John A. B. Allan's "Identification and Treatment of Difficult Babies" in *Canadian Nurse,* 1976, 72 (12) pp. 11–16 with the permission of the author and the journal.

Contents

Conclusion

To the Parents

The birth announcements have been mailed, the presents received, the first joy and excitement are now over, and reality is setting in. You have a new baby—not a doll, or toy, or something imagined, but a real, live, active, squirming, demanding infant. What to do? Most parents dream great dreams for their children. How do you start trying to make these dreams come true? Most likely you've had some preparation, at least for handling the baby's physical needs, but how do you proceed beyond that?

This book is offered to help you and your baby off to a pleasant start. The research on infant development in the last ten years or so highlights how very important this time of life is, and how very important you are in influencing your child. Your child is like no other. Your role involves learning about the special qualities of your child, and in *Baby to Parent, Parent to Baby* we'll look at how you can spot and nurture these qualities. Your baby is also like all other babies in some ways, and here, too, our knowledge can help. For example, all babies obviously need sleep, but not all need the same amount or sleep at the same time of day. All babies obviously need to eat and to have their diapers changed, but you will find that your baby will be unique in how often and in what pattern these events occur.

A basic part of parenting in this first year is learning about your baby, and using what we know about all babies to help your own. There *are* parenting skills, there *is* knowledge about infants, and then—to put it all together—there are *you* and *your baby.*

What do all babies need? From the moment of birth they need some one person or some very few people to provide them with consistency of care in a loving and responding way. They also need stimulation—exposure to the exciting world of people and objects, natural and man-made, that surround them. But this consistency, love, and stimulation should be matched to their own tempo. This book suggests ways you can make the match.

Although I have observed hundreds of babies and their parents, I am impressed anew each day by how much babies can do, and how aware they are of the important people in their lives. They are born human—not molded into humans. They have special human abilities, built into their bodies over the centuries, to help them survive and learn. Smiling, crying, and responses to language sounds are very early signs of this special human quality. Although helpless to meet his or her own basic needs for food and physical care, your baby comes equipped to get and hold your attention—and to build a loving relationship with you.

By following certain patterns, you can help your baby achieve a positive approach to the world during the first year of life. I call these patterns the Four P's. They are not mysterious scientific tricks of the trade; many parents show these patterns without naming them. But by becoming aware of them, you can do more of them, enjoy them more, and share them with others who may help you care for your baby.

First, there is *Ping-pong.* You know the fun of a long volley. It takes two to play, and the more skilled each is, the more fun. Ping-pong with your baby is a different form of the game. When you play with your baby, there's no competition—you both win. The object of a back-and-forth activity with your baby is to keep the volley going. The book will give examples of Ping-pong as an informal, joyful momentary event you'll want to repeat often during the day. The volley may consist of play, or simply of smiles, words, touches—any exchange between you and your baby in which each shows attentiveness to the other.

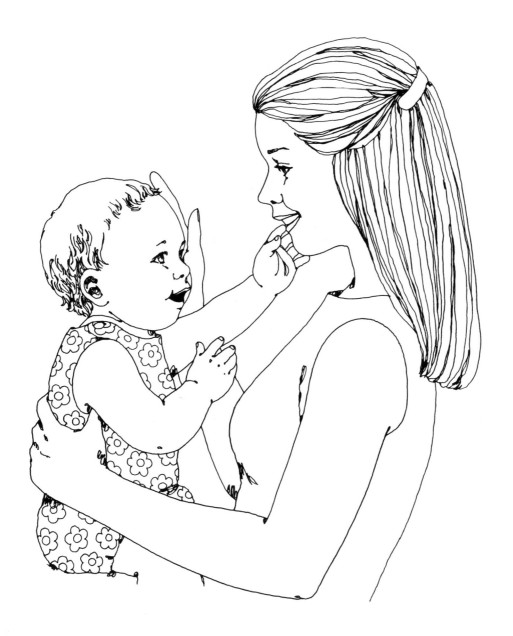

Second, there is *passion*. You know the thrill of looking into another's eyes and seeing a response. Parent-baby eye-to-eye looks are basic to building the ties between you. These begin very early, even in the first hours after birth. But passion is more than eye messages at a distance. You and your baby need to hold each other, to feel each other's warmth. Your baby's message is not "look, don't touch!" but "look and touch!" The book will give you some examples of ways to increase mutual contact.

Third, there is *perseverance*. Even in the first year of life,

3

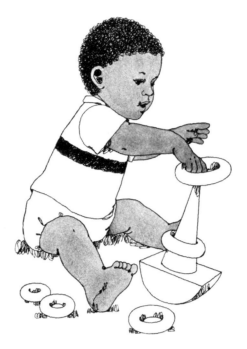

babies are busy checking out what's going on around them. They explore with eyes, hands, feet, and mouths. They need time to do this on their own. It's surprising how long they will stay with something that interests them. Parents need to learn when to back away and let the baby be. The child's perseverance is an important ability that, while somewhat influenced by his or her own body, is either encouraged or discouraged by what parents do and provide for the baby to do.

Fourth, there is *patience.* Sometimes this is in short supply; we've all been taught to "count to ten." There is evidence that we should all count at least to three (slowly) between the time we've signaled a person to do something and the time we step in again, and we should give another count of three of the time between a person's answer and our response. Think of a slow-motion Ping-pong game, rather than a fast, hard volley. Matching your behavior to your baby's unique rhythm, finding just the right beat, the right tempo, takes time and practice.

What do the Four P's add up to? *Responsiveness.* You can play Ping-pong, show passion, allow the child to persevere in certain activities, be patient and set a pleasing pace once you know yourself and your baby, and know in general how all infants develop. This book will give you clues to knowing and enjoying your baby, to letting the baby enjoy you and the world— to uniting loving and learning in infancy.

Before the Baby Comes

Once you've discovered that a baby is coming, the marriage relationship changes. You'll both need to make plans, think about your feelings, voice your wishes and fears. Just as conception is a joint enterprise, so is the prenatal period. The more you share the experience with each other, the more likely it is that your baby's arrival will be a joyful event; the more likely, too, that you'll be able to meet your growing child's needs for stability and continuity of care.

You can begin by:

SHARING HOPES AND FEARS

Does it matter if it's a girl or boy? Why? What do you expect of a baby? How do you feel about discipline and behavior—loose or tight? What worries you?

SHARING FOR SHARING

What do you see as the proper role of mother? Of father? Should both be equally involved, as work schedules permit? Who gets up for the inevitable "night shift?" Will you both handle the chores of changing, soothing, stimulating?

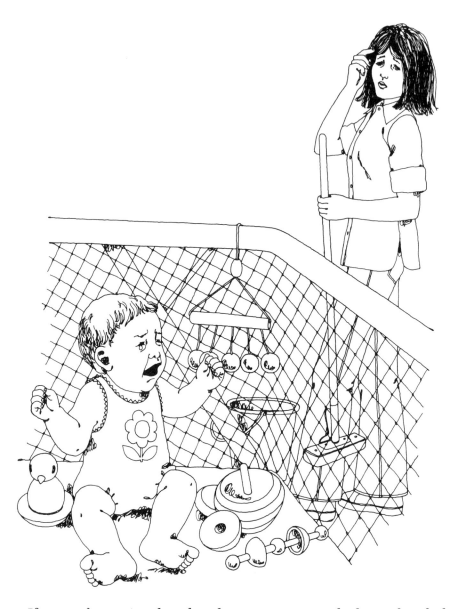

If you haven't already done so, now—before the baby comes—is the time to work out some of your sex-role ideas, so that a new partnership emerges.

But there are some preparations only the mother-to-be can make.

EATING RIGHT

Diet is important: what you eat affects your baby's development. Be sure you eat a balanced diet. (No doubt your doctor will have specific suggestions along these lines.)

Avoid *all* drugs, even aspirin; stop smoking, if you haven't already stopped—or at least cut down. Watch all those extra cups of coffee.

The father-to-be can help by curbing his habits so that your temptations are reduced. It's no fun to see another indulge while you deny yourself.

CULTIVATING SERENITY

Since anxiety increases the need for calmatives or cigarettes, a vital partnership role is to provide support, reassurance, and as smooth an environment as possible. It is particularly important in the last three months of pregnancy that life be tranquil. Some research indicates that a very anxious or stressed mother may have a fussier, more high-energy baby. Of course, all women are somewhat anxious—as are their partners—in the last weeks before their babies are born. But avoid added strain.

PLANNING TO BREAST-FEED

Preparation for breast-feeding should begin when the pregnancy is about four and one-half months along. There are a number of suggestions for preparing your nipples so that the baby's sucking will not hurt. If your doctor can't give these to you, a local La Leche League can, or you can do the following:

> Wash twice daily with soap and water. Use little soap, and be sure to rinse well. Use a soft cloth. As your nipples get used to it, change to a rough cloth. When your nipples are adapted to the rough cloth, move on to a soft brush and then to a hard one. After each washing, apply cream, petroleum jelly, or moisturizing cream to the breasts and nipples.
>
> If your nipples are flat or inverted, you should massage them. Grasp the nipple between your thumb and first and second fingers, pull it gently outward, and then massage.

Don't overdo—stop when you are slightly uncomfortable, don't persist until it hurts. Be regular about it; make this preparation a part of your daily routine.

But more than physical preparation is important. As you know, breast-feeding has sexual and deep emotional meanings that go far beyond the special values of the mother's milk. How do both partners really feel about this? How will it influence your relationship? What will it mean when it's 2:00 A.M.-feeding time? Is it a private or public act? Again, now is the time to plan and work it out, not at the last minute and not as a one-person decision.

PREPARENTING

You can also prepare by taking over the care of a relative's or a neighbor's less-than-six-months-old baby for several hours. Not only will this give your friend or relative some time off, it also will give you a chance to experience the energy demands a baby makes and have some sense of the responsibility of care. The period should be long enough for feeding and changing. That will give you some idea of what is ahead for you.

But don't panic if you haven't worked all this out in advance. Sharing, planning, and cultivating serenity are acts you'll continue long after the baby is born. There will be daily opportunities for these. Also, having the baby will create needs and opportunities that you can then use to work out feelings, roles, and relationships as issues emerge. What is most desirable is steady and open communication.

No matter how much you and your partner plan, your baby's arrival will still be a peak event, changing your lives in unpredictable ways. You will change as you help your baby develop and grow. Your dreams will be changed by the baby's reality, as they should be, so each day is an experience in growth for all.

There are other plans to make—space and equipment you'll need to prepare. Further on in this book I offer some suggestions for carriers and safety.

Birth—One Month

KNOWING YOUR BABY

Your first act as a new parent will be to make sure all is well with the baby. First you'll probably look at and touch the arms, legs, and body. Then you'll test to get a response, either by eye contact or by voice. Even very young babies, in the first hours after birth, respond to human speech. They spend long periods in a quiet, alert condition, relaxed, with eyes wide open. This is a good time for you to seek a response. This section will give you ideas you can use at such times, to see how your baby is doing. You can see by the infant's responses how ready the baby is to learn and grow.

But a second part of knowing your baby is to observe his or her temperament—the set of remarkable and early signs of the infant's own individuality of rhythm, activity, and awareness. Since what you do often is in response to some action of your baby's, knowing these signs of individuality may help you relax and enjoy each other, rather than place you in a battle of your general views versus the child's specific patterns. Building your child-caring patterns to mesh with your baby's own temperament not only will enable the baby to thrive, but also will take some of the pressure off you and promote harmony rather than discord.

Check-out counter. The first few days offer you many opportunities to know your baby's readiness and individuality. Your physician often uses a set of standard actions to discover readiness, but you can use them too for your own discovery. As you see your baby make responses to your actions, you come in touch with each other. Don't approach these acts as "clinical"—you are *not* diagnosing your baby. See them as teaching you what your baby is about, and what your baby can do.

Blow in my ear. The gag line "Blow in my ear and I'll follow you anywhere" applies to infants, too. You can do this even the first time you hold your infant after birth. Whisper in your baby's ear when he or she is awake and alert. Often the baby will turn to your voice and, on seeing your face, establish eye contact. Then you can look into your baby's eyes and begin to establish the marvelous emotional tie between you. You'll see that your baby is not passive, but ready and able to be an active partner in this new relationship.

You'll discover that your baby can be soothed by sound, especially if it's of low intensity—not "heavy metal" rock music. Your voice is such a sound, and is perhaps the best soothing sound of all.

In the hospital nursery or at home, if your baby sleeps or stays in a place where you are not present, low-intensity sounds can help induce sleep.

The eyes have it. Babies learn much from watching what goes on around them, even if they don't always look as though they are responding. But they also show their awareness by responding actively.

Babies are able to follow movement, and what they seem most likely to track is a moving, talking person. If you want to see how much your week-old infant's eyes can do, so that you can then place objects (or yourself) where the baby can see and enjoy them, try this: While the baby is lying in the crib, lean over and smile and talk gently. It doesn't matter what you say. Then move to either side (just your neck and head), and watch your baby follow you.

Your baby will also follow a picture of a face. Try this: Hold the baby comfortably in your lap, take a picture of a face

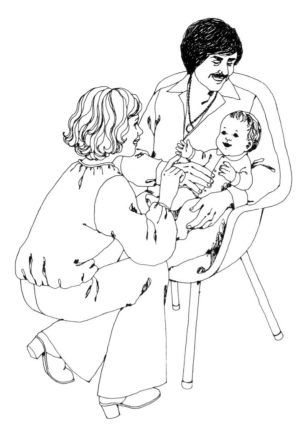

(with big eyes) and move it across the baby's line of vision. Of course, you should do this when your baby is in the quiet, wakeful, alert state, maybe just after being changed.

You and your partner can do this together: Let one hold the baby on the lap, and the other be the moving target. That's even better than placing the baby in the crib.

The oral zone.
Obviously, a primary need of the infant is food. Your baby comes equipped by nature to use his or her mouth to make contact with a source of food, and then to get the food. You already may have seen your baby use both the following techniques. You can make little touching games out of them—but, please, not teasing ones that may deprive your baby of the pleasure of accomplishment. And don't deny the baby food, or delay feeding, to try these.

While your baby is comfortable on your lap, gently touch the corner of the mouth and move your finger toward a cheek. The baby will turn head, mouth, and tongue toward the side you are stroking. Now touch the middle of the upper lip and watch the baby raise lip and tongue. As your finger moves up

11

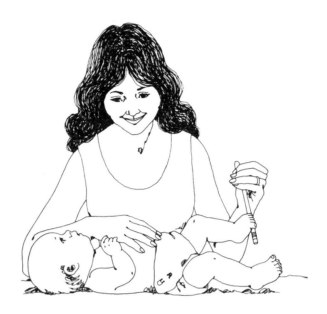

toward the nose, the baby's head will go up and back. If you place your finger on the lower lip, the baby's tongue and lip will go down, and so will the head. This is nature's way of helping the baby find the nipple, and it's called *rooting.*

For most babies, sucking comes naturally. Once they've found the nipple, away they go! But, for feeding to be pleasant, especially if it's breast-feeding, mothers have to be relaxed and comfortable, too.

Babies will also suck when no food is involved. You can place your finger gently in your baby's mouth and see this work. Usually by about three months of age, the baby will have replaced rooting with movements of mouth and head, and will also have discovered how to get his or her own hand in the mouth to suck.

Contact.
Nature also gives your baby ways to hang onto things when they are placed in either the hand or the foot. It's surprising how strong your baby's grasp can be. One easy way to tell is to place a finger in the baby's palm. She or he will grasp tight, and you can raise your baby's head from the crib or bassinet.

12

If you place a finger in each palm, your baby will open the mouth and close the eyes while grasping your fingers. This, too, is a strong grip. The baby will respond this way for a few months, gradually replacing this involuntary natural action with more voluntary efforts to pull upright.

Your baby's foot also shows the tendency to grasp. This is not as strong as the hand grasp, but will occur if you press your finger (or a pencil) just behind the toes. Watch the toes try to curl to hold your finger.

If you want to see just the big toe flex and the others fan, rub the end of your finger (easy does it!) along the bottom of the baby's foot, starting at the heel and going toward the toe.

All babies usually have these responses. If your baby doesn't seem to respond, it may be the way you've tried, it may be the time of day or the baby's state (tired, hungry, etc.), or it may be something else about your baby. The best bet is to talk it over with your doctor, who has more careful and controlled means of seeing how your baby is doing.

Sometimes the baby's hand-mouth movements, rooting and grasping, get in the way of feeding. That is, when the baby is placed in the feeding position in your arms, the baby's hand comes to his or her mouth. The hand is in the way of the nipple.

This can be a time for *Ping-pong*. Have your baby grab your finger (placed so that it is easily reachable) and have a hand-to-hand game going while you get mouth and nipple together. You can accompany the action with soothing words and sounds.

This is also a great time for *passion*. Your baby, even if only a few days old, will search for your face while feeding, and you can get eye contact. The warmth of being held, the satisfaction of feeding, and the comfort of an easy solution to hand-in-the-way all give your baby and you a good start.

ONE OF A KIND

You are well aware there's never been another baby just like yours. That's true because of the way human biology works. Each of us is special, not only because of our genes, but also because of prenatal care and conditions and what hap-

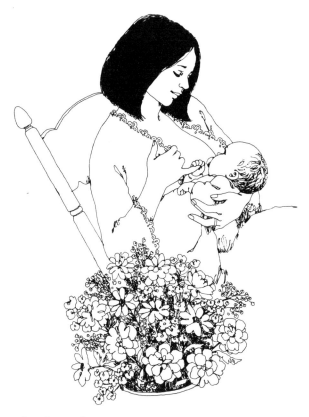

pened during birth. What are some of the ways you can see this specialness, beyond the obvious ones of fingerprints and other detective-story clues?

Sex differences.   As the French say, *"Vive la différence!"* Boys and girls do differ from one another, and not just in outward appearance. Probably the first question you asked after finding out that your baby was alive and well was about the baby's sex. Whether they are surrounded with pink or blue nontraditional colors, children's behavior from birth on is influenced by their sex. That means there will be a tendency (with a *lot* of leeway) for certain patterns of behavior to occur. What are these?

Although scientists are not all in accord about how much these differences are biological and how much they are due to learning what society expects, it seems to be a fact that generally boys are more aggressive than girls and have more muscular strength. They also seem more predisposed to learn through visual and spatial means, while girls seem more predisposed to learn through oral and verbal means. Girls are also likely to smile more often. However, in the first year of life these dif-

14

ferences are minor. Both girls and boys will pay about equal attention to sights and sounds, and certainly both will put everything possible into their mouths to taste, test, "gum," and chew.

In the first few days, a boy baby may cry more when hungry, and take a little longer to be comfortable; girls may be more alert and aware of surroundings when feeding.

But being aware of your child's sex should not cause you to place him or her into a behavioral pigeonhole. If your baby is a boy, he's more likely to deal with you at a distance, but he'll also need and enjoy being cuddled and hugged. Your girl baby is more likely to respond to your words and your touch, but she may also be strong and aggressive. The key to knowing your baby is making your own observations and then using what you see in order to reach and communicate with him or her.

Temperament.

Activity level. Perhaps the easiest way to see how newborns differ is to compare your baby with the others in the nursery. Babies differ in wiggling, getting their fists to their mouths, sleep movements, rate of breathing, and hardness and rate of sucking. It's not that one rate or pattern of behavior is "good" and another "bad." The important point is that the child's own activity rate affects the demands on you. Put that together with your own activity rate, and you'll know what you need to watch. You may be a deliberate, easy-paced person with an active, vigorous baby—or the other way around. If you like things to click right along, speedily and on schedule, a low-activity baby may have trouble fitting your style.

Observe your baby's behavior when the infant is home with you. He or she is still getting used to being out in the world and is inconsistent in behavior during the first few days in either the quiet, wakeful state or right after feeding. Activity rate while sleeping seems more stable. You can see close at hand what you observed in the nursery.

Rhythm is tied into this. Each of us is better at some parts of the day than at others, and we need more or less sleep than some of our friends may require. These differences emerge early—and you can see them in your baby. There are three main cycles: sleep-wake, hunger, and elimination. While there are "averages", and the so-called typical baby will sleep about sixteen hours a day in the first few weeks of life, no baby is "average." *Your* baby will have his or her own rate for each cycle.

During this first month, adapting to the baby's cycle rather than expecting the baby to fit yours, helps build the beginnings of your baby's trust in you as someone to rely on. Not that your baby knows who you are! Babies just know that life is comfortable—things happen to fill the tummy or remove dampness without much waiting or crying and fussing. Adapting to your baby's rhythm is *not* "spoiling," but being responsive. The pattern will be obvious to you if you look for it. It's easier for you to follow the baby's pattern than to try to get the baby to follow yours.

Intensity. Some of us go at things harder than others do. Some babies cry harder, suck harder, push harder, grab harder, just seem to "put more into it" than other babies. There is probably, as in most things, a middle ground—between very intense and passive—where babies are easiest to live with. A "difficult" baby may be more intense than you expect—and may drain your own energy—or nonresponsive to your efforts, not intense enough.

What can you do? You can't actually change your infant's intensity of response; you just have to cope with it. If you see early that your baby reacts vigorously to feeding, changing, and play, and seems to get red-faced and fussy before eliminating, you can perhaps be calmer in your approach. Your calmness will help to make the relationship smoother, though it will not necessarily reduce the intensity of your infant's response.

Charge! Retreat! How do you feel about going into new situations? Are you a plunger—ready and eager to go? Or do you hang back until you have the situation "cased?" Do you avoid the new, feeling good mostly with the familiar? While some of your pattern was influenced by your experiences, some of this inclination to charge or retreat was present very early. Your baby, too, will reveal early a tendency to approach or withdraw from the new. This may not be easy to see in the first month but will become so as the baby is introduced to new foods, new people, new objects and toys. The reaction can be mild or vigorous, but you will know. An early sign is the baby's reaction to being bathed.

Your baby's style will become more important after the first month, and I'll make some suggestions about it in the next chapter.

Happiness is . . . . Babies differ in mood. Some do quite a bit of cooing, gurgling, smiling, and a little later, laughing; while others seem unhappy and are more likely to cry or be fussy. Of course, the happy baby is easier to live with, and you may want to spend more time with the infant because you're having fun. If your baby is not so happy, you may have a tendency to be unhappy in reaction—to fuss at the baby more, or let the infant "cry it out," or just find ways to put some distance between you. That's natural. But the unhappy or fussy baby probably needs your positive response more than the happy baby does. So you have to look at your own feelings, and learn not to get angry—your baby is not crying or fussing purposely to annoy you—but to help the baby be comfortable. Here is where passion, especially rocking, holding skin-to-skin, and singing or making rhythmic sounds may serve. It may not make your baby "happy," but it will give you both a chance to share a pleasant time. It may also help you handle some of your feelings. *Patience, perseverance,* and *passion* on the part of the parents make the positive approach.

Awareness of the world. Of course, all new babies have to learn about the world of people and objects. Some, however, seem more aware of what is going on around them than others do. Some seem to be influenced more by what is going on in their own bodies. In the first month of life, all the major activities of the baby are tied into bodily demands for survival— food, sleep, warmth, elimination describe the daily (seems like hourly) round. But on top of this, your baby is also getting to know you and the world, even though he or she cannot tell people apart, or really "think."

There are several ways babies differ in getting to know the world. We have already mentioned Charge! Retreat! But babies differ in how easy or hard it is to attract their attention to voice or sight or touch. They differ in how easy or hard it is for them to fit into their parents' schedules and routines. They are unlike each other in their ability to stay with something—to persevere—and they differ in how easy it is to distract them, to shift their attention from one activity to another.

Your child's blend of all these differences—activity level, rhythm, intensity, mood, and the like—is further proof of his or her uniqueness. The child's patterns in each of these areas of difference will now become visible to you, and during the next two months will become even more distinct.

As you get to know these regular patterns of sleep, reaction to events, feeding, mood, you can not only adjust your views and actions to suit them, but you will also become alert to changes in the patterns, signs that the baby is "not himself" or herself. These may mean stress or infection and may signal a call to your doctor or a closer look on your part at what you are doing.

USING CARETAKING AS LEARNING AND LOVING TIMES

You don't have to set up special times of the day for observing your baby. The usual caretaking routines provide plenty of opportunities.

Feeding, changing, bathing, getting to sleep and waking up—the quiet, alert times all give you chances to see your baby's patterns, and to respond in a consistent, loving way. Loving and learning in the first month is mostly *your* loving and *your* learning about your baby.

As you meet your baby's needs, he or she begins to learn about the world and will begin to learn to love the parents who have provided a good start.

Some things to do—when.

Feeding should be a source of pleasure for you and your baby. Babies suck not in a constant rhythm, but in bursts. They suck, pause; suck, pause. A baby who is not on the nipple (breast or bottle) during a sucking time swallows air, and that hurts! Watch your baby, and help him or her by getting nipple and sucking response together. The newborn at the breast may lick the nipple over and over before sucking.

A baby also can be distracted from feeding by stimulation. Although stimulation is necessary, there are times when it gets in the way. For a pleasant nourishing time, stimulate (stroke, hold finger, talk) when your baby is at the end rather than the beginning of a pause, not during sucking or when a pause is begin-

18

ning. Proper timing seems to prolong sucking, insuring a fuller meal, with less air, in a shorter time. This not only assures your infant of good nutrition in a comfortable way, but also makes feeding a less taxing time for you. Long feeding times, with burping and discomfort, tire you as well as your baby.

Crying is the infant's way of telling you something is wrong. What to do? How fast should you respond? You can soon tell what the cry may mean—hunger, uncomfortable temperature, wetness. See it as a signal. Since a baby can know you are tuned in only if you do something, a glance from a distance to be sure that the blanket isn't caught doesn't tell your baby anything. Try to respond fairly rapidly, even if you are in another room. Make ninety seconds your outside limit. Think how fast you go to answer the telephone: ninety seconds is fifteen rings!

Generally, the best first response is to pick up, hold, and cuddle your baby. This may stop the crying, and then your baby's eyes may open and you can gaze at each other.

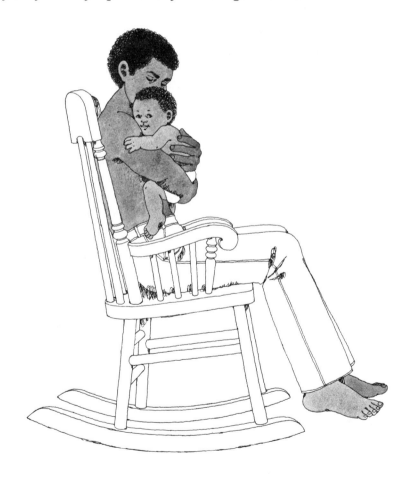

If the baby's calmness is only momentary, feeding is the next step (assuming that you've already investigated changing). If that's what the signal was for—as you can soon predict by noting your baby's rhythm—feeding should be followed by relaxation and sleep.

Some babies, however, don't respond to being held or even to being wrapped warmly. If your baby is fussy, and cuddling, change, and food don't work, try a continuous low-pitched sound. In certain cases, running the vacuum cleaner is a sleep-producer!

Some babies tend to respond to several things at once—rocking, holding, and soft singing all together may soothe them. Babies can respond to the rhythm of your voice as early as sixteen hours after birth. There was (and is) a lot of sense to the old-fashioned rocking chair and lullaby.

Fast and appropriate' response—whatever stops the crying, soothes the baby and you—is *not* spoiling your baby. It enables his or her body to thrive, actually cutting down on the baby's need to cry to signal you in the months to come. It begins to build the child's sense of trust in you. Not answering, rather than stopping the cry, increases its length and intensity (till baby may stop from exhaustion), gets you tense, places you and your baby as adversaries ("That baby is *not* gonna run me!"), and sets off a downhill cycle.

But everything in moderation. You can't always use the less-than-ninety-second rule, and sometimes it seems that in spite of everything you do, your baby is still crying. Don't worry if occasionally you go overtime. It is natural for there to be times when you and your baby are out of tune with each other. Remember, your less-than-one-month-old infant is influenced more by what is going on inside the skin than outside. You are more a responder than a starter. Your baby doesn't know you or know that you are trying to care; so the infant is not trying to bother you, but simply trying to satisfy bodily needs.

If you can't get the baby to stop, give your partner a turn (you should be taking turns, anyhow) if more than one adult is home. Some babies are hard to read—you can't easily tell what's bothering them. The way you are responding may be what's provoking the baby. In any case, try not to turn it into a contest. Another person, at that moment, might be more relaxed, and somehow a baby senses this. Calling time out and sending in the substitute should occur before you sense yourself getting angry at the baby, or at yourself.

Some of this assumes there is a partnership arrangement. There may be two parents, but no worked-out ground rules for sharing infant care. That turns the baby into the football, and the adults may be opposing teams. A parent needs relief, needs time out, needs the physical support of another. When your baby is crying, and life looks overwhelming, and energy is low and temper high, that's no time to work out parental roles. Don't turn your baby's crying into a battle cry.

Sleeping. When people tell you that babies sleep sixteen hours or so, that doesn't mean *your* baby will, nor does it tell you what his or her cycle will be. There are also stages of sleep—from deep sleep to almost-awake. Babies may open their eyes while sleeping, and you may well confuse this with their being awake. The best bet is to assume that if your baby is awake and needs you, she or he will let you know.

The main concern during this time is safety. A crib should have slats narrow enough (less than two and three-fourths inches wide) so the baby's head cannot get caught. Don't tie a pacifier or any other object around the baby's neck. Don't put in the crib or tie to the crib objects that might accidentally be swallowed or somehow choke or smother your child. Remember, babies move and kick during active sleep. While generally a baby will automatically work to free his or her face from a smothering blanket, it still poses a hazard. If the crib is safe and you don't hear from your baby, you can assume all is well. This lets you do whatever else needs to be done, or get your rest. You may be anxious if all is too quiet. A visual check is enough. It's okay if the baby moves, or makes faces, mouths and sucks, or even occasionally seems startled. No need to disturb the baby's sleep. You'll appreciate your chances to rest. Sleep becomes a cherished thing. Don't disrupt the baby's or yours if you don't have to.

If your baby's breathing seems irregular, or if your baby's face seems different than usual, then you may wish to make a closer check, and let your doctor know.

Learning by looking. Your baby will spend some time in a quiet or active waking state. This is a good time for cuddling, talking, or carrying the baby around. It's a time for eye-to-eye contact. Babies learn a lot from looking, so give your baby things to look at. You can place colorful pictures on the walls. Dangle (at a safe distance) a mobile over the crib, since your infant will tend to follow its movement, at least for brief moments. Babies seem to prefer patterns, and yours, too, may enjoy and watch pictures of faces more than just unpatterned, even colorful, objects. Don't go overboard: if there's too much clutter, your baby may block it out by going to sleep.

When you carry your baby around, make sure that he or she can look at the surroundings. The choice of carrier should allow for comfort, body contact, and visibility. The best ways are in your arms or in one of the new soft canvas carriers. However, some babies, when cuddled and comfortable, become drowsy and don't get much looking time. If you notice this, you may sometimes want to use the kind of carrier that is detachable from you, or another type in which your baby stays alert.

How you get the best mix of body contact and alert state is very personal. Again, you are the keenest observer of your baby. Babies need both touching and looking time. But some babies, at some times during the day, may prefer that you look—don't touch!

The alert time offers you many chances to start a game or exchange with your baby. The other "whens"—feeding, crying, changing—require you to respond to the baby. Now *you* can be the starter, and your baby will enjoy responding to you. You can pick up the baby, smile, talk, stroke, and rock. This is the time for Ping-pong and passion, independent of caretaking. Just be sure your baby's responses show you that the fun is mutual.

During this quiet, alert state, your baby can also amuse herself or himself. That is why the pictures and mobiles are useful. In another few months, your baby will coo and babble pleasurably when alone. Just like you, the baby needs a mixture of social time and private time. Hovering is not helping.

Changing. Unfortunately, there are parts of child care no one particularly enjoys. Babies do wet and have b.m.'s, and they need to be cleaned and changed. In spite of the TV commercials in which women are shown happily discussing what brand of diaper to use, these are usually the low points of the day. Our way of life requires infants to be diapered, and we also expect homes to smell clean and be sanitary. With all the disposable products, it may not be the laundry burden it was, but change time is usually seen as nothing but a chore.

22

There's no reason this cannot be a shared activity. A man has enough finger dexterity to change diapers, and, strange as it seems, changing the baby may bring him not only physically but also emotionally closer to the baby. Seeing your own baby nude, especially if changing is turned into a playtime, may have a powerful, positive effect.

Your baby will be in a wakeful state, and you can try this: After your baby is cleaned, and before putting on a diaper, lean over and smile and make low, pleasant sounds. You can accompany this with a gentle tummy rub. Your baby will most likely respond by waving arms and legs. You can then pick up and hold your baby skin-to-skin, and, supporting the head, let him or her look around while being firmly held. You can then place your baby on the changing surface, and try for mutual gazing. This makes changing a chance for Ping-pong and passion. You can also use this time for check-out.

You may find, and don't be surprised at it or misinterpret it, that your boy baby has an erection. Don't get scared, or feel

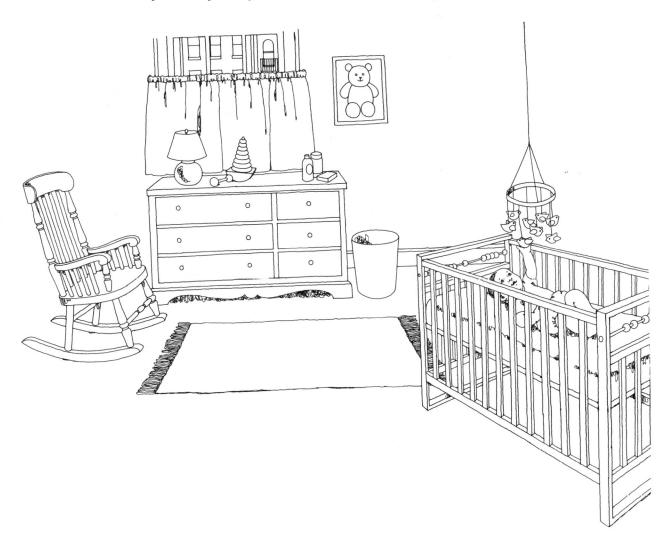

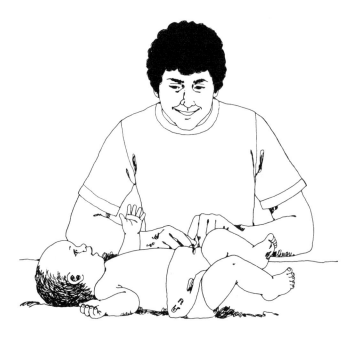

you've done something to stimulate sexual arousal. It's a natural event, and will also happen during sleep or in the bath. He is just being a boy; he is not depraved, nor are you, for holding and cuddling your baby.

Bathing. Another opportunity for active exchange with your baby is during bath time. Most babies enjoy the warm water, the contact of parents' hands. Of course, they don't like soap in their eyes, or washcloths over their noses, or other acts that cut off sight or breathing. As in changing, fathers can and should share in this routine. The other suggestions for eye contact, soothing sounds, skin-to-skin fit in here too—after your baby is dry and not slippery.

During this first month, there are many chances both during routine care and at alert, awake times, not only for you to come to know and enjoy your baby, but also for your baby to begin to know and learn about you. This first month is a busy time for both parents and infant. Parents also learn much about themselves and each other, as a baby requires new patterns of behavior from them. It is a time when your baby begins the most important activity of the first year of life—building trust in you, herself or himself, and the world.

Responding to your baby's individuality and providing consistency of care helps all of you off to a good start.

24

The Second and Third Months

One of the delights of having a baby is watching the rapid development that takes place in these early months. Sucking, rooting, grasping are reflexes a baby is born with. Your infant does them without thinking about them, most likely without even knowing he or she is doing them. In these months, more of your infant's behavior will be due to things learned in the first month's experience, as well as to built-in (maturational) patterns of development. Actions will be more likely to occur because your baby wants them to—he or she will be actively trying to do things. There is always the danger of thinking that infants know more than they do (they *don't* think like us!) or ascribing to them more will power than they have. But these months are the time when your infant begins to be more social, more aware of what is going on around him or her.

There are important attitudes and feelings that have their beginnings in these months. One is the development of trust, which follows up on your responsiveness in the first month. A second, begun now but continued probably throughout life, is the discovery of selfhood. Each of us is aware that we are separate individuals. In some special sense, each of us is alone. We have a private part of us, deep down, which we do not share even with those closest to us. The discovery of our individuality can be frightening, or it can be exciting and challenging. At the same time we are becoming aware of our own separation from other people, we are also finding out that these other people can be nurturing, supporting, loving, protecting, stimulating.

One-month-old to three-month-old babies obviously are not thinking about all this, but it is happening to them. Your infant's developing abilities are equipping her or him for developing selfhood. The experiences you provide during this time can work in harmony with your baby's development. You can assist in the creation of both trust and a positive view of self.

Many scientists are looking at how parent and baby communicate with each other, and how that affects what they call "attachment." This is the desire of each to be near or with the other, and, later on, the knowledge that one can count on the other. Adults with positive views of self recognize when they can do things on their own, and when they need to rely on others. As the prominent British psychiatrist John Bowlby has shown, the healthy, self-reliant adult has had, since early infancy, experiences that have taught her or him to have both trust in others and trust in self. This seems to rest upon the development of attachment in infancy, beginning in these first months.

SIGNS OF DEVELOPMENT

Rather than describe the obvious gains in height and weight, let us look at what in your infant's behavior shows awareness of the world, readiness to learn and respond, and ability to communicate needs and feelings.

What's going on? Your baby's behavior will show that she or he is asking that question by the use of eyes, ears, mouth, hands, and total body. *Learning by looking* continues. Your baby will look around more. He or she will spot and "track" a moving object if it is not too far away, first by following it in a straight line horizontally, then, about a month or so later, up and down, and then a week or so after that, in a circle. Your baby will show a preference for moving over fixed objects, for three-dimensional over two-dimensional objects. He or she may prefer red and blue objects over gray ones, and bright over neutral tones. About a third of the quiet, wakeful time will be spent in looking around.

But your baby is also learning by looking at herself or himself. She or he will start to watch her or his own hands as they flutter into view. Toward the end of the third month, your baby will be making efforts actively to view the hands. Moving objects are more interesting than fixed ones—and ones he or she can move and control (the hands) are even more fascinating! The baby who is active and intense may also accompany this effort to watch his or her own hands with grunts, feet wiggling, and general body movement. Everything seems to be going at once, but you can see the main effort is in exploring the hands by means of the eyes.

Your baby will try to find out what (or who) is making sounds. He or she will begin to connect your voice with where you are in the room.

Babies' increased ability to control their heads and trunks help in increasing their use of eyes and ears. By the end of the third month, most babies can lift their heads to look around when they are lying on their backs, and can lift their chests. This enables them to look around, connect sights and sounds, and explore their environments.

Along with increased head control, there is an increase in the ability to get eyes, hands, and mouth all working together. The coordination is not very smooth, and will get "polished" only in the next several months. Before this coordination, when your baby grasped your finger or anything else you placed in his or her palm, there was little if any effort to bring the hand to the mouth. Now you will start to see the "testing by tasting." *Everything* gets to the mouth! Indeed, by the end of these months, or early in the next three months, your baby will probably open his or her mouth as though in anticipation of getting into it any object he or she sees close at hand. No wonder Freud called infancy the oral period! The mouth is the baby's most sensitive area for learning by touching, and it gets used to the full. It is not that your baby is either being "cute" by using the mouth; nor is your baby willfully disobeying your "no-nos" and physical efforts to stop her or him when potentially dangerous or dirty objects head for the mouth. It's just that infants learn through how things feel in their mouths—and this learning begins now.

This object-to-the-mouth routine is also another way your baby learns that he or she is something different from the people and objects around the crib. Not only do foreign objects get mouthed, but also the baby's own body. Sucking or mouthing one's own hands has a double sensation—in the mouth and on the hand. This is one way your baby discovers that the hands belong to him or her, but that the nipple or other object does not. Sucking on the bottle or mother's nipple gives one type of pleasurable feeling in the mouth. Mouthing hard objects gives another feeling. Foot-in-mouth, a harder trick that comes later, also helps your baby get a notion of what is part of one's own body. If you see these acts as evidence of your baby's growing ability to sort out the world, you can relax and enjoy them—provided you've kept unsafe things away.

GETTING TO KNOW YOU . . .

In these months, babies become more aware of people and events. They show this increased social awareness in several ways. Your baby lets you know that she or he anticipates being fed by making sucking and other mouth movements when you come into view for feeding. This action shows that your baby has learned to connect your presence at certain times with being fed.

Your infant also shows by changes in activity, facial expression, or type of movement that he or she can tell the difference between people and objects. Usually by the end of the third month, a baby knows the difference between Mother and other people, and responds differently to her voice and presence. Some babies seem to be able to do this as early as one month. Timing probably depends upon both their own temperaments and the amount and type of experiences they have had. There is no reason to push for this recognition, since all normal babies will get there before they are six months old. It is just another sign of individual differences.

My use of the term "mother" here does *not* exclude father or other major caretakers. Most studies have observed infants and mothers. As more fathers share in child-rearing and as more infants are cared for by non-family members, we can predict awareness and attachment to them. Indeed, we know that

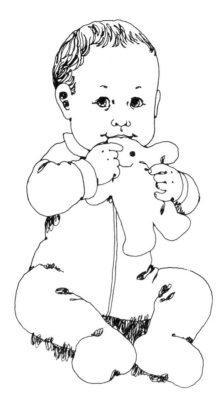

infants can be attached to several adults, although the tie to one is usually more intense.

The same behavior that tells you your baby knows that people are different from objects, and that Mother, Father, or principal caretaker is a special person, also shows that your baby is beginning to realize that he or she is a separate person. Babies do this by reacting to being left alone, picked up and put down, passed from person to person.

During these two months, infants will most likely protest being put down. Indeed, the high point of such protesting (fussing, crying) is just before three months of age. Some infants begin to protest being left alone in a room about the second month of life. Objecting to that grows with age—at least throughout the first year of life. For most babies, being left with others does not cause protest until they see parents as separate from other adults.

Infants show their awareness of people by smiling when someone smiles at them. The social smile, brought on by eye contact and smiling, is a fascinating event for the parent. This becomes even more exciting when it is clear that your baby knows you—and is smiling at not just anyone, but at you! This is a strong element in building attachment. There is nothing quite like it—except your baby's first word. It shows that she or he is aware of and is in special contact with you.

See what I can do! A basic part of being human seems to be the desire to have an effect on the world. We all, to some degree, try to influence what is going on around us. We learn and tend to repeat those actions that show us we've had an effect. Our folklore and literature are full of slogans telling us how to control or change the behavior of others. We've all read, "A soft answer turneth away wrath," or "Do unto others. . . ." Your baby too, being human, will start to show you that he or she enjoys affecting the world (you and objects), and is more likely to learn when the world responds.

You have already noticed anticipation—mouth open, ready to feed—as one sign of learning. Attentiveness to your presence, to voices, is another sign. Your baby is tuned in to you, because your response to his or her actions tells your baby that he or she has the influence needed to cope with the world.

Your baby is *beginning to solve simple problems:* "How do I get Mommy or Daddy to come?" "How do I get that mobile to rattle?" "How do I get that thing in my mouth?" But the response doesn't always have to be from you. The infant discovers that he or she can do something better this week than last. The perfection of motor skills—getting the body to do what the infant wants—is very satisfying and enjoyable. That is why your baby spends a lot of waking time in motor acts. The baby is not only learning where self ends and the world begins, but also what power he or she has to make his or her own body and the world respond. Your baby discovers and enjoys these activities in which his or her own actions have an effect. Maybe that is why hand- (and later thumb-) in-mouth lasts so long: your baby has found an enjoyable act that she or he can do at any time.

What is stimulating is not simply the presence of objects or people, but the connection the baby discovers between his or her actions and the actions of the people or objects. Actions that show your baby that he or she can make things happen are powerful and stimulating actions. What is happening is that your infant is taking inborn actions—rooting, grasping, sucking, looking, listening—and is putting them together. He or she is making combinations of acts. Grasping and looking and suck-

30

ing, for example, go together in the object-to-and-in-mouth pattern. Although the movements are awkward, practice will make them smooth and efficient. Your infant will practice not only because both the result (getting whatever-it-is in the mouth) is pleasurable, but also because the sense of increasing skill is so satisfying. Out of such actions both competence and the sense of competence are built.

Your baby is growing in capabilities in yet another way—expressing *feelings*. At about two months, your infant will begin to be able to let you know that he or she is happy. Up to now, your baby could communicate discomfort by crying and fussing, but had no clear way to express pleasure. Cooing, babbling, strings of vowel sounds, and then the social smile all are outward signs of delight.

Your baby is still more skillful at expressing distress than at expressing happiness, but that is probably because your baby is still so helpless to take care of his or her needs. Letting you know that he or she is uncomfortable is essential for survival; letting you know that he or she is happy (at this age) is not.

Up to about the end of the first month of life, your baby's crying was primarily a distress signal, meaning hunger or pain. The so-called colicky baby's cry is irregular in volume and pitch. It has a tendency to irritate the hearer. The more usual cry is more rhythmical. But during this period your baby will develop a new cry—a signal for attention. It's not clear how you can tell the meaning of your baby's cry, but most parents can tell hunger from pain. The attention-seeking cry, while not as crucial for physical survival, is nevertheless important. Remember the baby's need to have an impact on the environment? Remember that your baby is also beginning to learn that you are separate from him or her? Put these together and you can see that an attention-getting cry is an important signal. It *is* a cry for help. The help needed is not food or diaper change or sleep. The help needed is to know that you are there and will come when called. It may be seen as a need for trust and security.

Your baby will also express unhappiness by fussing, whining, whimpering, or by stiffening in your arms. These signs are like words to you. Watch when they happen, and they will tell you about your infant's development. They may happen when you separate yourself from your baby—putting her or him down in the crib is the best example. If you understand that these are the only ways your baby has to convey unhappiness, you can react in a more relaxed manner.

Since your baby can't speak and has limited ways to express feelings, he or she may express them more forcibly than you expect. This is especially true of negative feelings—anger, distress, discomfort. They may tend to "turn you off," but they are part of your baby's survival kit—they are built-in ways to get action from you. Your responding to them helps your baby go on to more mature and less irksome ways. Your failing to respond may lead to their stopping by exhaustion, but that doesn't help your baby grow. Responding by scolding or punishing, letting out your anger or frustration, may not only increase the crying and fussing, but also may teach your baby negative lessons. Communication is a two-way street. Not only is your baby learning to let you know how she or he feels; your response teaches your baby what you see as the right way to react. He or she learns that while you will respond, your punitive response increases discomfort. Your baby may learn that the world is not a comfortable place. He or she may also learn that through strength and power one imposes and controls another. That is probably not what you meant to teach at this early age.

These two months offer you not only chances to learn about your infant as you did in the first month, but also opportunities for influencing your infant's development in learning and loving. There are things you can do, always remembering that your baby is special, to help make family life more pleasant and to provide ways for your baby to use his or her increasing capacities to deal with self and world.

THINGS TO DO—NEW EXPERIENCES

Baby-sitting. When can you go out and leave your baby with a stranger? Sometimes there is a tendency to be too protective of your first baby. That is the path to exhaustion and frustration. Brief separations are not disruptive, but prolonged separations between the ages of four and twelve weeks are not desirable. Your infant is working on attachment and has learned (although he or she is not necessarily showing it) to expect certain behavior from you. Your baby has found that certain of her or his actions will bring actions in return from you. A long break in that developing routine should be avoided. A few hours out won't matter; a weekend away might.

Even if you go out for an evening (and you should), briefing the baby sitter is important. Your substitute needs to know how you play the game. Show and tell your baby sitter how you respond to, hold, handle, coo at your baby. Show how you make diaper change a Ping-pong game. Try to create for your baby a situation that remains consistent even when you·are absent.

Consider developing a cooperative relief/sharing group in your neighborhood, if there are other parents with young babies. A cooperative is especially useful when you plan to be away briefly. Other new parents are most likely to appreciate your needs and those of your baby, and you can enjoy sharing ideas in a small group over the coffeepot. And you'll save money, or be able to go out more often. Cooperatives are less useful if a long separation has to occur, because another family may not be able to assume the responsibility of long-term caretaking.

Although a long separation (several days) may not be expected or planned, emergencies happen. It is good to have a back-up plan. Find someone you can trust, and show her or him your pattern. Let your baby become familiar with the person; even take your baby to the other person's home. Begin your baby's "familiarity training" early so that if anything comes up during the year, you have a way to cope. This is important for all babies, but especially so if your baby's temperament requires special understanding. Try to match caretaker and baby—find out the caretaker's attitudes, rhythm, and activity level so that you don't invite care problems.

The outside world. These months are ideal to not only show off your baby, but also to introduce your baby to the world. Because your infant learns by looking, take him or her our for chances to look around. Your baby will probably find it interesting and exciting to be held in your arms or close to your body in a carrier—especially with head up and with no obstacles to looking—while surrounded by the color, movement, and noises of street and shop. The baby will feel protected, but also will be able to explore through eyes and ears. If it's too much, your baby can also turn it all off by going to sleep!

Going out of the house also exposes your baby to many people, some of whom will come close and "ooh and ah," or try to touch your infant. You can determine how close to let people come. Holding your baby firmly will let the baby know whether you are relaxed or tense. It's probably better in these months to let others establish eye and face contact but to maintain a little apartness. Babies are remarkable—they can let the stranger know whether to come in closer or not. A lifted arm with palm open suggests a "shake hands" contact; a look away means "Keep your distance." You can see these signals and feel them in your infant's body. Follow his or her cues, and relax.

Remember *Charge! Retreat?* Your baby may not respond comfortably to new experiences. But she or he does need exposure. Babies need to become familiar with the world. You may have to go easy, but don't take what looks like the easy way out, staying at home and sheltering the infant. You can best show your love by helping the infant learn to adapt to new settings and people by introducing them in a comfortable, relaxed, nonpushy way. You will need to hold your baby so protection and reassurance are communicated by body contact.

New foods.

Sometime in these two months your doctor will suggest that you introduce new foods into your baby's diet. Good nutrition is a tremendously important base for good growth and development. Your baby's brain, for example, is going through its most rapid growth in this first year of life. If you are nursing, your milk remains the best, most nutritious source of food available. If your baby is on formula, then your doctor will suggest whatever changes need to be made. The physician will often recommend the introduction of solids but will not necessarily say which ones, or how to help your child learn to eat them. The easiest approach is to buy prepared foods. But check the labels—these are often very high in sugar (That's why babies like them!). A better approach, even though it takes more time, is to prepare the food yourself. It doesn't take much strength or time to mash a banana or squash green peas. Where possible, do it yourself and cut down on both cost and sugar.

Some babies enjoy being introduced to new foods and are eager, easy eaters. Others don't like change. Just look at yourself: is your diet fairly limited and consistent, or do you vary it

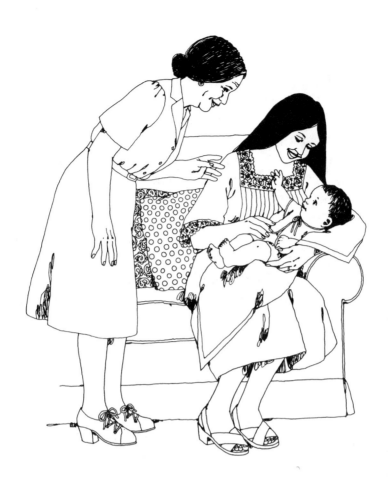

a lot? When you eat out, do you go to the same old place and order the same few dishes, or do you try new places and sample new foods? Your baby won't starve if he or she initially rejects new foods. A gradual introduction is fine. Try variety until you find those that he or she likes—and preferences may lie in texture, color, smell, or taste. Babies can thrive for a long time on milk and bananas and vitamin supplements! Don't make an issue of it.

Approach the introduction of new foods as you would approach any new experience for your baby. Watch your baby's reactions. Bring passion and Ping-pong into play. You can make sounds, model a wide-open mouth, smile and laugh between your baby's mouthfuls. Mealtime should be a social time, devoted to enjoyment of each other, not a struggle to get food in. The baby's attitudes toward you, toward food, toward self are all wrapped up together and formed by how these times are handled.

THINGS TO DO—AT HOME

The daily grind.
Every day has its routine. Many who seem to have the best and most interesting jobs will report on how much· of their days are not exciting or eventful. Special moments are usually few. That's true at home too. The excitement of caretaking is offset by what can become drudgery. Feeding, diapering, bathing, etc., can become routine. Further, since your baby sets the pace (particularly for changing diapers), it can be like having an impulsive and demanding boss. This is why all parents need some "time out." But there are ways you can increase the pleasurable moments and even turn the dull ones into chances for loving and learning.

After eating, your baby now may not go right to sleep. He or she will stay alert and awake for longer periods of the day. This is a time for play. Play is a vital way for children to learn. At this age, of course, your play with your baby is not through organized activities or games, but may be just body- and eye-contact sports. Giggling, talking at, laughing, stroking, tickling, lifting, and vigorous rocking are all forms of parent-infant play in these early months. Your baby's response will tell you what the limits are. Many babies, when hunger needs are met, want stimulation—and you are the best stimulator. This search for activity will increase during the first year, but it begins in the second month. Human beings like excitement. Your baby doesn't seek or enjoy the dull daily routine any more than you do.

But you can't be, and shouldn't be, with your baby during all the time he or she is awake and playful. In parent-infant games, there is a difference between playing with your infant and interfering. You should respect your baby's rights to be alone, to be separate from you.

You can however, rig the crib so that your baby can learn by looking and doing. I have mentioned the use of pictures and mobiles. Now you may mount a cradle gym so that your baby can bounce and get it to jiggle, or try to grab one of the gym-rings. These crib fittings help your infant work on putting eye and hand together, on building skill in getting the environment—which in this case is the cradle gym or mobile—to respond to his or her acts. This is fun as well as educational.

It is no substitute for you, for human interaction, but it is a

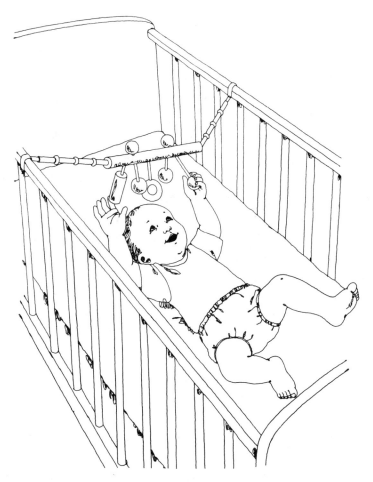

supplement. It is possible, as has been done in many laboratories, to so rig a crib that babies get "turned on" for long periods of time. It is easy to tie one end of a string to a baby's toe and the other end to a rattle and see that a baby soon learns to make the rattle move by moving the tied toe. Cribs have been rigged so that babies will play records of their mother's voice. These are important ways for laboratories to learn about infant capabilities. It doesn't mean that you should go overboard for gimmicks at home. There are, first of all, safety considerations. Strings can get loose and be swallowed. They can also somehow get around a baby's neck and cut off air. Stick to the simple, safe things. More than that, getting a baby hooked on gadgetry is not necessarily useful for good *human* relationships. So while it may be tempting because your baby will find it entertaining, don't overdo the crib bit.

The discovery that a baby, given a chance, will select to listen to his or her mothers' voice shows not only that a baby can learn and can control the string to get the recording, but also that his or her truly basic want is mother's voice!

Words. convey love. Your baby doesn't yet understand your words, but the rhythm, tone, and pitch of your voice does register meaningfully. Even in the first month, babies show (by listening and looking more), that they find a parent's face and voice more important than a stranger's.

How do you help? During caretaking, you can talk gently to your baby, pausing as though in conversation. You can ask questions (even though you'll get no oral answers) and use your voice to show pleasure or excitement. What you say is not so critical as how you say it. Babies will show they are listening and attending by their eye, head, and body movements. Conversing is different from lecturing—which is one-way talk, usually of an informing or ordering nature. Listen to yourself when you are trying to explain something to someone, and when you are just having a conversation. There's a difference in emphasis, loudness, and rate of speech. Your baby can tell this difference too. What's needed here is the light touch—you are not teaching, but holding a dialogue.

You can talk to your baby even when you are at a distance. You can be doing the many chores that have to be done, and your baby can be awake in crib or bassinet, or in a blanket on the floor. You can talk informally, describing what you are doing or just making chitchat. This type of talk at a distance seems to help babies feel less uncomfortable with strangers later, when the babies are about nine months old. If you provide your baby now with exposure to words, people, objects at a distance, your child is likely to be more relaxed at nine months, when virtually all babies go through a "fear of strangers" time.

Vocalizing, making vowel sounds, begins now, during the second and third months. As I've suggested in *Baby Learning Through Baby Play,* there are dialogue games you can play. While you're changing the baby, he or she is likely to make an "ooh" or "ah." You can ooh or ah back, smiling and making eye contact. What happens? Baby oohs, you ah, and an ooh-ah Ping-pong volley is set off. You can also move your head in closer when it's your turn, and your baby will move toward you. It's both a vocal and a body-movement game. It can go on for quite a while, so be sure you are in a comfortable position when you start. I've played this form of Ping-pong for as long as twenty minutes—till my back gave out!

This type of vocal sport can go on at any time during the

38

day, during just about any caretaking procedure, and can be started by either your baby or you. It's a great way to build attachment, because it capitalizes on that special human ability—the ability to talk to each other.

HANDLING DISTRESS

One of the problems all parents face is how to cope with a baby's discomfort. Since you will have begun to recognize the differences between pain and hunger cries, you already have some ways to handle your baby's needs. But sometimes feeding doesn't lead to relief, or being checked for wetness or a jabbing safety pin or the like doesn't solve the problem. Sometimes babies are just plain distressed, and physical child care is not enough. As you now well know, babies differ in how much pain or discomfort they can handle, how much need they have for help, and how they will use or resist help.

Early in these two months, soothing through holding, cuddling, vocalizing, and gentle movements seem generally most useful. As your baby gets closer to three months of age, stimulation seems to be more effective. It is almost as though the younger infant is distressed by what goes on inside his or her body, and your helping lies in restoring the body to some level of comfort. The older infant, being more aware of the environment, can be calmed by increased rather than lessened activity.

Rocking is a good example. Gentle rocking, along with firm holding and soft sounds, is useful for the one-month-old. Even "overriding" the baby's cries with a steady, louder sound (remember the vacuum cleaner) helps. Some have found that swaddling the baby (wrapping tightly in a blanket) is comforting and sleep-producing.

At three months this begins to change. Vigorous rocking seems to become more helpful. You may want to equip a crib with rockers instead of wheels, so you can give it rapid pushes (about one a second)—and push with some force. No guarantees, but both the rate and force seem to go together to help distressed infants. You can try this, and see for yourself.

Rockers on the crib also allow the infant to rock himself or herself, and you may hear this in the middle of the night. Not

39

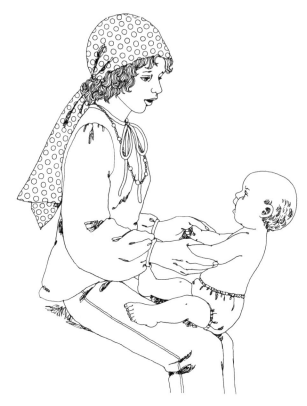

to worry (but take a peek). This is another example of how the infant will use his or her body to get the environment—here, the crib—to respond in ways that are pleasurably exciting or soothing.

THE "DIFFICULT" BABY

Some infants need even more help in coping with distress, and various holding techniques have been found useful. Again, you know your own baby, and you can watch both the baby's and your responses to each other. You can tell whether your baby needs more than the usual activities given above. The two procedures below have been extensively adopted from psychologist John A.B. Allan's work with parents of "difficult" babies.

If, by about the second month, your baby is whiny and especially irritable and can't seem to relax even in your lap, then you might try this: When your baby is in one of these irritable states, sit down and hold the baby loosely yet firmly in your arms or on your lap. It is important to hold the baby's arms and hands in your hands and not to let go until the baby

40

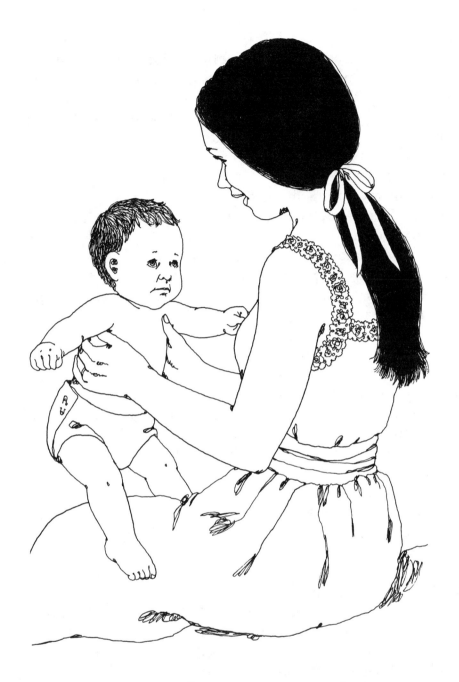

is relaxed. If the baby stiffens and tenses, gently increase your pressure until it is slightly greater than the baby's, so that her or his arms and legs respond by bending at the joints into a re-laxed position. This will probably result in a rage response from your baby, followed by more extension of limbs and stiffening. During the rage, keep the baby in your arms or on your lap, and give her or him a movable barrier to rage against. That is, *do not* let your hands and arms act as a straight-jacket type of

41

restraint, but keep them firm enough to provide some flexible opposition. When your baby stiffens once again, apply gentle pressure to a point sufficiently strong to reduce the stiffening. Most likely, there will be another rage reaction. Continue as above. After a few minutes, your baby will probably begin to sob.

Now relax your holding and begin to comfort the baby and to encourage the sobbing. You can do this by the tone of your voice and by tilting the baby's chin to his or her chest. After sobbing, your baby may fall asleep for a while or lie contented and relaxed in your arms. In some cases, it may take several cycles of the rage-sobbing-relaxation pattern before the baby experiences prolonged relaxation. On the average this can usually be experienced in ten to thirty minutes. It is very important that a satisfactory end state of relaxed attachment between parent and baby be achieved. Incorrect holding (allowing the baby's legs and hands to disengage or become detached from yours) will result in a longer, low-intensity struggle and lead to a shorter period of relaxation.

This might take you a half-dozen attempts, but it will help your baby express tension by real crying (with tears) and/or by rage—and then your baby will be able to be cuddled and relaxed on your lap.

The "stiff" or "rigid" baby, one who tries to fight free of you, can be helped by these actions: Spend five or ten minutes holding the infant up—that is, lifting the baby from underneath both arms and keeping the head slightly forward—moving her or him up and down, back and forth in space while you face each other. Smile at your baby. Most babies cannot resist this type of stimulation. Even if in the midst of a rage reaction, they will start to smile and chortle. With *perseverance* in this approach (doing it whenever you want to cuddle your baby but find him or her stiff and rigid), you will find that your baby's muscles will relax in time.

Some babies show such extreme forms of muscular tension that the release that comes from smiling and laughing is only temporary. If you find this so, you can move your baby's body about, like an accordion; that is, you can open and close the arms and legs gently and rhythmically. Your baby will most likely get angry and cry, but this will lead to relaxation and attachment. When sobbing starts, help it by comfortable holding and by making sure that the infant's hands and feet are not crossed over each other or touching each other. Usually the rigid baby has his or her hands gripped together and legs crossed over. Once again, in time and with perseverance in this approach, the rigidity is reduced, the baby becomes more sociable—you'll see more smiling and cuddling behavior—and consequently the need to use this type of holding diminishes. The baby will now respond to normal parenting practices and interactions.

At other times of the day, when your baby is in the crib, you might try placing the infant on his or her stomach. That way there is something to push against if your baby needs an outlet for all that intensity of activity. You might even put the force to positive use by placing an interesting mobile in such a position that your baby can see it best when he or she has pushed up and has the head high.

Most babies don't need the above two holding measures; always use the least restraint and effort you can. These are emergency techniques, or actions for some babies.

What you have to do is put ideas that seem to work with other babies together with your own experience with your own baby and find, by trial and error, what seems to work for *you* and *your baby*. But always keep in mind that *you* are the one able to think, and try to solve the problem. Your infant can signal to you and respond to you, but can't solve the problem on her or his own. Your baby's distress bothers you—but it also bothers your baby! It is not done deliberately to provoke you.

There's the poem in *Alice in Wonderland*:
Speak roughly to your little boy,
And beat him when he sneezes:
He only does it to annoy,
Because he knows it teases.

That may be okay for the Duchess in Wonderland, but not for you and your baby in the real world.

Much has gone on in these two months as your child's awareness of the world has grown. You are building the pattern of attachment and trust between you as each of you learns about the other and the ways to relate to each other. But development, especially in this year, is rapid and brings not only new pleasures and new dimensions to the family relationship, but new challenges as well. Let's look at the next three months.

From Three to Six Months

The last half of the first six months is one of rapid growth in your baby's awareness of the world, and ability to maneuver in it and to communicate with it. Brain development is rapid, so your baby can and does learn many new skills in these three months.

One way to look at what takes place is to use the word *mastery*. Your baby will use these months, and of course those that follow, to get a firmer grip on both body and world. Actions will be more controlled—you will see some primitive planning—rather than just being responses to the immediate environment or to bodily needs for food and comfort.

Your baby, in other words, becomes a more organized person, able to make arms and legs do more of what he or she wants—and do it better. Babies are now more able to stimulate themselves, more able to take in, through eyes and ears, what's happening around them. By the end of six months of life your baby is more adept at getting around by his or her own motor power. That's a lot to happen in a short time. The rate, of course, is different for each child, which is why there are no tables of weekly achievements in this book. Don't use the month estimates I provide as rules, but as guides.

And remember that there is another whole area of learning. It lies in your baby's learning to feel good or bad about other people, and about himself or herself. When your baby reaches a milestone—such as rolling over from tummy to back, or creeping, or sitting up, all of which provide far more freedom to see and do—how do you respond? What would happen if you were to ignore the achievement, or let the baby know either that it's not much and you expected more or that you are sorry to see the baby move away from you? What would happen if you were to fail to provide the baby with the new experiences he or she can handle? Your pattern of nonresponse or negative response would inhibit your baby's practice of the new skills—and the joy in them. Part of the fun of doing new things is to hear the cheers of the crowd. Shakespeare taught us "all the world's a stage." The baby sees himself or herself as star actor and wants the attention and applause! Your enthusiasm will help your baby develop self-esteem. Just as the baby needed (and still needs) response to cries for help, so he or she now needs response to new successes.

Fortunately, most of the time parents feel good about what their baby does. They view new skills and actions as favorable signs of growing up. They see each period of time as having its own excitement and neither push the baby for more nor try to hold the baby back.

The baby's mastery of new skills, then, requires not only the biological development that usually comes as part of being human, but also support, help, and frequent responses from parents and other caretakers. Mastery is another aspect of self-reliance, and it depends on attachment and love as much as on physical growth.

SIGNS OF DEVELOPMENT

I can do it!   Control over the body is a major development in these three months. You have been able to prop your baby up—usually in one of those plastic cradle-boards or carrying boards—for a while, but your baby couldn't do it for himself or herself. More than that, such propping often restricted head, arm, and leg movement. (I'm generally against such devices, but some parents tell me they are useful at times.) But now, by the end of the fourth month or so, your baby will enjoy sitting—and can sit, with some support—on your lap. Head and back control now enable the child to do this. Sitting on a lap is so much better for loving and learning than being propped up in plastic or against pillows! Your baby still very much needs your touch, and his or her increased head and back control give both of you opportunities for physical contact on your lap—with less restraint from fear of falling. By the end of six months, a baby can usually sit in a chair alone, and the high chair or "Baby-tenda" now offers more utility and freedom to observe.

The inborn grasping ability (remember you tried this?) should be gone, but it is replaced by controlled behavior. The infant will practice and grow quite skilled in reaching, grabbing, and holding. (See *Baby Learning Through Baby Play* for some games to play.) Sometimes these activities will get in the way of diaper-changing or dressing, because your baby will want to reach, grab, and hold the diaper or clothing while you are trying to change or dress that moving target your baby has become.

A major locomotion development begins at about four months. Try this to see it: Place your baby tummy down on the floor. With head held high, your baby will make "swimming" motions, using arms and legs, and work hard at moving forward.

"Swimming" will be followed, about a month later, by actual creeping. Your baby can now use hands and knees and tummy to get from place to place. That *is* a major social and physical event! It creates a whole new set of opportunities for your baby and you.

By six months, your formerly nonmobile baby can now sit, roll over, and creep; reach, grab and hold. Since a basic fact about human beings is that they will practice and use any skills they get, your baby will want to do all these things—sometimes when you don't want them done. These new motor abilities can lead to clashes between you and your baby. The "Things to do" section will deal with these. A good general rule is to give your baby the least restrictive environment you can, always with safety in mind.

Listen! Language learning also takes place during these months. It has two parts—learning by listening, and learning by vocalizing or making sounds. Just as babies learn by looking, without making any response we can see, they also learn much

46

about language by listening before they can talk. In these months they become more able to find the source of a sound. Even though, of course, they can't see the sound itself, they can turn toward it. This may not seem like much, but think what has to go on in the child's mind. He or she has to hear a sound, figure out that it is being produced by something somewhere, be aware that what is producing it is *not* visible, and make the connection that, by turning one's head, one can find the source. That really is a remarkable achievement for a four- or five-month-old! Further, the three- to five-month-old responds by organizing the body to pay attention to the sound. He or she is likely to stop an activity, widen the eyes, and then start another activity that leads into the searching for the source. At six months, listening and searching are the major responses.

These are essential steps in language learning, because for the very young child, language equals attentiveness to others' speech. If your baby doesn't seem to follow this pattern, it would be wise to have your physician check. It is hard to detect hearing problems in infants. One way is to see whether your baby, in the regular daily routine, shows alertness to sound and tries to find its origin.

All these new skills enable the child to learn at a distance. Since we live in a world of space and have to figure out how to judge distance and size, these early skills are vital. Experience with objects, people, and sound at a distance provides the infant with the basic ingredients for making his or her way in the physical world.

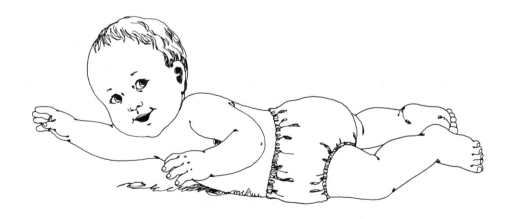

Your baby's increased awareness of sound and speech, along with the new motor ability, opens up more communication opportunities for the two of you. For example, since your baby can roll over and sit, you can, when dressing the baby, say "Roll over" while you help her or him roll over, demonstrating what the words mean. This way, action and words get put together in the child's mind. You can lift your infant's leg, and at the same time say "Lift your leg" so that the child's voluntary actions get connected to your words. You may find that you have to occasionally use "Hold still!" But that, too, is part of growing.

Call your baby by name, or nickname, when you talk to her or him. Your name is a very important part of you, and the same holds true for your baby. During pregnancy, you thought long and hard about possible names for your baby. Now use the name you chose. Although your baby cannot recognize his or her name, this will come in a few months. But it can happen only if *you've* used the name in talking with or playing with your baby. Don't use it only when you're upset or angry—in harsh and loud tones. Be sure to use it in pleasant tones at pleasant times.

Self-stimulation.
The baby's self-stimulating actions increase during this time. Now he or she will be able, at will, to get thumb or toe in mouth. That is one form of self-stimulation. There are three ways babies stimulate themselves: by mouthing, by using their fingers on their skin, and by rubbing their bodies against sheets, blankets, or anything else handy. When do infants do this? And why?

The first reason is: just for sheer bodily pleasure. The skin is an erotic zone; the mouth particularly is sensitive, and serves also as a source of information about the world (objects are hard and soft, warm and cold, fit and don't fit); movement through rocking or being rocked is arousing as well as at times soothing. The search for bodily pleasure seems to be basic, and shows up very early in life.

Mouthing is very common, as I've said before. It takes many forms, with sucking of hands, fingers, and thumbs, and various lip movements the most common. Sybille Escalona, a prominent child psychologist, was able to count thirty-one different mouthing patterns in sixteen- to twenty-week-old infants!

It doesn't seem to be connected to pleasure or distress—many babies use sucking for comfort, others don't. Those babies who tend to be inactive may be most likely to mouth when they are comfortable and relaxed.

Since mouthing and sucking are so natural for infants, there seems to be little reason for parents to keep pulling fingers out of infants' mouths, saying "No, no," or getting upset. Mouthing *will* go on during this time and will persist for quite a while. If you think of this as a part of your child's development, one that, once satisfied, will be abandoned for later and better means of learning and comforting, you can relax. You wouldn't think of stopping your infant from creeping because you are afraid that the enjoyment of creeping will prevent him or her from ever standing up and walking. You know that babies "outgrow" creeping and that it's a necessary step in learning to walk. Look at oral activity in the same way—as a necessary step that meets infant needs. Watch adults—they still mouth in many ways, but no adult (that I know about) is still sucking a thumb!

When in distress, babies will scratch, rub, pinch, or pull at and poke their own skins. When babies are very hungry or very tired they often scratch or poke—and kick and fuss while doing it. It is not clear why this happens, but certainly it doesn't promote calmness. It seems that when very uncomfortable or in pain, even adults tend to hurt themselves. It is as though self-induced pain somehow overrides or minimizes the pain one can't control.

Since this self-injury happens when the baby is very uncomfortable, your early response to cries and other distress signals may lower the amount of time he or she feels this way, and thus reduce your baby's need to "beat up on" himself or herself. Lessen the discomfort you will feel at witnessing such behavior by attending quickly to your baby's discomfort.

Babies also stimulate themselves by body contact with sheets, blankets, and the like. Perhaps most often the baby will roll over or back and forth in the crib. Rolling is a self-starting act that your baby enjoys when awake, alert, and comfortable. (Rolling just the head is probably a sign of fatigue.) This action will be infrequent now, but it will occur more often in the next few months.

Mouthing and rubbing actions show the increased control

the baby has over his or her own body. More and more often now, your baby will be seeking and finding ways to get pleasurable sensations through mouth and skin. You can provide some ways in your touching and holding, stroking and grooming acts.

Just look around you. Watch how often we adults stroke, pat, groom ourselves. Babies are not another type of human being; all of us, unless taught otherwise, seek bodily stimulation and use it for soothing and for pleasure. If you learn to look at your baby from this vantage point, you'll be less worried or upset by your baby's normal ways of soothing and satisfying his or her body.

Communicating.
These months expand your baby's social world. The increases in motor and brain development enable your baby to do and learn more, and to be more aware of you and what you do. This is a time when individual differences in activity rates can be particularly important influences in development. The passive or inactive baby is more likely than the active baby to need you to start the action. The active baby is more likely to seek you out, to begin the Ping-pong game, to let you know that he or she wants to play. When the baby is around five months of age, social transactions not connected to child-care activities will increase considerably, then stay fairly constant. In our observations of videotapes of mothers and infants, made at the Institute for the Development of Human Resources every six weeks, beginning when the infants were thirteen weeks of age, my colleagues and I found that social exchange, especially mutual gazing into each other's eyes, was highest between four and six months, and that the amounts of it also influenced how a child performed on developmental measures of thinking and response to language at one year of age. It was from these observations that we developed the term "passion."

This social contact also has its "discipline" side. Since the baby is able to do more things, he or she can also get into more mischief. Parents are more likely to begin or increase compelling, scolding, restraining behavior, and the infant is more likely to respond by resistance to such treatment. This most likely happens during child-care times when your baby moves around, making it harder for you to feed, dress, or change him or her. This can either be escalated into conflict, or can, by use of play and patience, lend itself to "détente." How you deal with the baby who now seems to make life harder for you depends upon your view of yourself and your baby. If you see the wiggling and attempts to move as normal development, you can cope. If you see these as threats to your authority and control, then there's trouble. There is no way to avoid moments of differences between what you want to do and what your baby is busy doing. But babies do need stability, order, and regularity, even though the rules of family life come from outside their own biological patterns and needs. How you create this stability, order, and regularity—whether by force or by a calm series of steps in response to your baby's growth and that matches your baby's individuality—is an important element in your child's self-development. This means that you don't suddenly come down hard on your baby, but that you match your requirements to the ability of your baby to respond to them. This takes trial and error, there is no easy way. When you see you are creating problems for you and your baby, back off—the baby can't.

On the wholly positive side, your baby will imitate some of your actions and vocalizations, will show delight by smiling and cooing as you play, will enjoy and seek social stimulation.

Your baby will even enjoy roughhousing. We found, somewhat to our surprise, that six-month-old babies laughed and enjoyed being held, lifted up, and wiggled in the air, even by an adult who was a stranger first seen only a few minutes earlier! The joy of the act overrode the former sober expression as a stranger approached. Of course, the babies' parents were right there with them. Remember, wiggling does not mean shaking in the way you would a salt container or a pair of dice. Easy does it.

We also found that children were unhappiest when placed in infant seats, even with favorite toys. People are more fun, more stimulating, than gadgets and objects.

Since this is a time—around six months—when babies actively recognize their parents and have discovered that there are differences in people, most respond differently to a strange person than to a familiar one. But, for most babies, that response is not a fearful one if the stranger doesn't rush at them, handle them too soon, or behave in a strange way (such as being silent—adults usually say *something* to or at the baby). When approached too rapidly, most babies simply get more watchful and sober. You need to alert strangers to the child's territorial boundary—the extent to which they can approach without some behavior by the baby that shows permission to touch or come nearer.

With a lot of experience with other people in your presence, your baby is more likely to trust new people. Just show, by voice, smile, or the way you are holding your baby, that they are all right! You have to think about how trusting you want your baby to be. In this world not all strangers *are* friendly. Your child is simply learning, in these early months, about two groups of people—familiar and new—and that is enough to handle. In the next half-year, he or she will begin further sorting out of people. This, of course, will be based on your baby's experience and your bodily and verbal cues on approaching or avoiding strangers.

Remember your child's pattern. Some children will seek out new experiences and people; others will resist or shy away from them. Match your exposure and efforts to the needs and comfort of baby, not to the words here about "most babies" or "some babies."

THINGS TO DO

What can you do, in the normal routines of the day and week, to foster the development of mastery in your child? You've seen your baby grow, during these months, in motor ability, awareness of people and self, and interest in things, people and events.

Your baby needs chances to use her or his new motor skills in a somewhat stable environment furnished with objects to see, handle, explore. Your first way to help is to be a stage manager, setting up the theater in which your child will be the actor.

Setting the stage. Since you cannot and should not be with your baby every moment of the day, you can arrange things to be interesting in your absence. Your baby will want a mix of new and old objects to play with. The fun toy responds to the baby's actions.

52

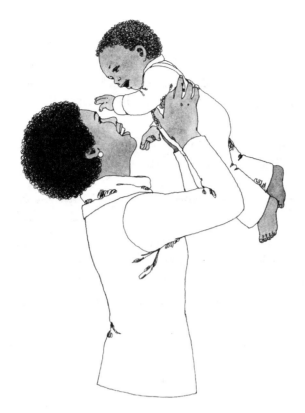

Look at your baby's crib. Can you redesign the mobiles and cradle gym for increased baby control? What will happen when your baby can sit up? Do things need to be moved for safety?

What can your baby see from the crib? Is the view interesting or blank?

Is the crib itself responsive? If it has rockers instead of wheels, your baby may begin to be able not only to rock himself or herself, but also to get the crib to move around the room. This can be startling, when you hear rhythmic bumps in the night, but it may be worth it. Later, when your baby can stand with support, he or she may be like a ship's captain, maneuvering the crib-ship all over the bedroom seas!

If movement *is* possible, be sure to baby-proof the area so that anything that can be reached, grasped, and placed in the mouth is safe. Again, beware of strings. If you use a pacifier, do *not* tie it to a crib slat or around your baby's neck. Your aim in using the string may be to permit your baby to reach the toy, but that string also can be (and has been) a noose.

Increase the chances for your baby to see, hear, converse (ooh-ah, smiles, and gestures) with both family members and strangers. Your baby is old enough to go places with you, from shopping to eating out, to car rides and visits to others' homes.

When boredom sets in, sleep is the usual way out. You may find that your baby gets "high" and overexcited from such trips, especially if lots of people make a fuss over him or her. You can work out a way to ration the activity or to time it to fit your daily rhythm and the baby's pattern. There's no point in your coming home exhausted and then trying to cope with an excited, eager baby who wants to play.

In the home, your baby's ability to creep and, at the end of this period and into the next, to sit up, requires many changes. *First,* you can involve your baby more (if you haven't already begun to do this) in the family's patterns. He or she can eat with you. If that's hard, at least have your baby near the rest of the family when you eat. Your baby will tune in to the conversation of your partner and you, and note the speech pattern, the back-and-forth flow, the taking turns, the tones and inflections that go with gestures. Although vocabulary is not yet being learned, the family's speech patterns are taken in. Moreover, your baby will feel a part of the family, increasing attachment, love, and security.

Second, your baby has entered the age of exploration and can now begin to go to things and people, rather than only have people and objects come to her or him. What a change! Try to arrange your space to help your baby use this wonderful development. Since the baby is much too young to understand safety rules or know that you value some breakable objects, it is up to you to "baby-proof" the space. You'll have to live with this adjustment a year or so, unless you want to spend a lot of time either restricting movement or scolding and otherwise punishing your baby. That's the hard way. Just as mouthing is na-

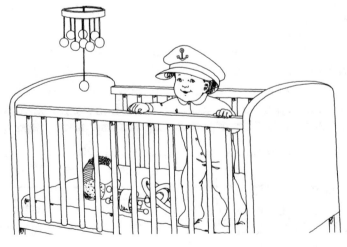

tural, so are creeping, handling, touching, and, a little later, biting and chewing.

What to do? Remember that your baby is more precious than material possessions. Put away, or out of reach, your bric-a-brac and souvenirs and fancy glassware. Your home is not a showplace, but a living and learning place.

You may want to cover the floor with soft materials, well anchored. You can also supply some low "targets" (stools, etc.) for your child to creep toward. He or she will later use these to pull up to and support standing. You may also cover good fabrics with protective cheaper, washable ones. Then you won't mind the occasional accidents of spit-up or leaky diapers or other events that can and do occur.

What about a playpen? If you can't be handy all the time to watch or if it is impossible to baby-proof everything, a playpen with good visibility may be a help. But be sure your infant has time out of it to "swim" and creep. The playpen does restrict movement. If you get a foldable one, your baby can be with you in safety, in the kitchen or out in a green area—park, playground, backyard. It allows your baby to be with you, to see you at a distance, but still to be occupied with safe toys to pull on, mouth, or grasp. Balance time in with time out of a playpen. You can see when it shifts from being a pleasant place to being a restricting one. Encourage exploration and movement.

Third, with increased awareness of you as a person and with increased bodily development, your baby will be more able to adapt to family routines. You can begin to organize the day more around your own cycle of meals, family time, bedtime. Your baby will be able to go longer between meals, and the baby's cycle can match yours. This is not an abrupt change of the rules of the game: you are still responding to your baby; you are not forcing the baby to respond to you. The change is gradual and two-way, and is heavily affected by your baby's development. Watch for ways to develop a family schedule, to build routine, all the while still responding to your baby's needs. This changeover won't be finished in these months. I sometimes wonder if it ever gets finished! Each of us has his or her own pattern, and family life requires compromise and adjustment. Your baby is least able of all family members to do this, but learning to do so can begin toward the end of the first six months of life.

Inactive babies will need more help. Setting the stage may not provide sufficient stimulation for the more apathetic babies. They will tend to use their eyes more than their other senses, and are also less likely to signal when they are hungry or distressed. And they are more likely to suck or rock or otherwise handle their own discomfort. Thus, it is easy to think of the quiet baby, who sleeps a lot, cries little, and is attentive to pictures or mobiles, as a "good" baby who doesn't require much attention. In fact, this is the baby who requires more, because the active baby will usually demand and get what he or she needs. Some see the quiet baby as "good" because he or she doesn't upset the old family routine as much. This infant lets you sleep more, do more of your usual things. But since he or she is neither demanding nor responsive, you can easily overlook the baby's social interaction needs. The inactive baby needs to be with people. Make a greater effort to vocalize, to help your baby handle and manipulate objects. Social play, Ping-pong, are *needed*—and you have to be the one who starts the games. You need to help your baby move away from the less mature pattern of attending to internal needs and body handling, and toward awareness and responsiveness to objects and people—the outside world. Your baby will not necessarily practice doing things without you. The cradle gym may go unused. The toys may not be touched, grasped, squeezed, and mouthed unless you set up the action in a lively play situation. The active baby will practice alone; the quiet one needs people to bring her or him out.

Person to person.   *All* babies need people. Setting the stage is only part of the drama. The more significant part is the action among the people. Even the active baby, who can practice motor skills alone, needs you. Only people can play Ping-pong. A mobile can jiggle when you move, but a toy or ball can roll out of reach. Even a responsive toy always gives the same response: if squeezed, it squeaks. Only people can match their acts to the baby's, moving in the rich pattern of give-and-take. Only people can add to this the hugs, smiles, words, and tones of voice that convey excitement, pleasure, delight.

.To see this, let one parent watch the other at play with the infant. Notice how both parent and infant move together, and how often the parent's move follows the infant's. Take a push-

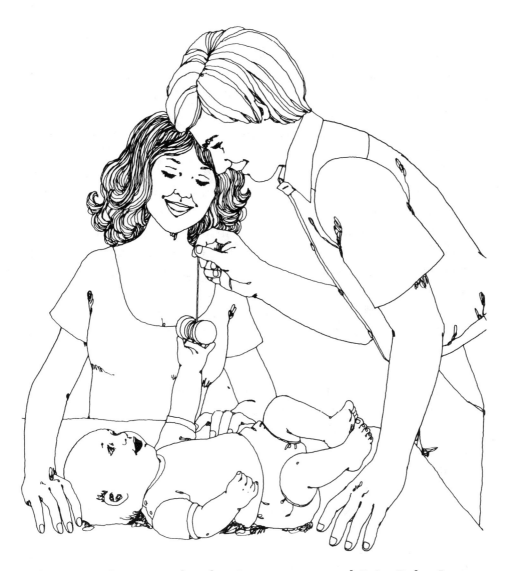

pull game (for example, the "two-way stretch" in *Baby Learning Through Baby Play*), in which an object is fastened to an elastic cord so that if the baby grasps the odject, baby and parent can tug and interact with each other. Watch how the parent gets the object close enough for the baby to see it, then reach and grasp. See how the parent helps and guides, using tone of voice and words. Its great fun for both and builds an intimacy no gadget can provide. It combines Ping-pong, passion, perseverance, and patience in a special responsive mix.

Trade off—have the first, active parent watch the other. There will no doubt be differences in tempo and style. But this, too, is what your baby needs. The infant will discover the differences between his or her parents and enjoy the special qualities and contributions of both. If only one parent is available, do this with a close friend who may be able to provide not only contrast but also consistency of care.

The dialogue (ooh-ah-ooh) becomes even more fun and useful in these three months. It seems to work best when there is eye contact. But you can also talk at a distance, when your baby is on the floor or in a playpen and you are several feet away but still visible.

Make use of your baby's developing ability to creep. Since your baby will want to be near you, let the infant follow you about like your shadow. Move slowly when you do this, because the five- to six-month-old is just learning and is not very skilled! You can also invent simple "come and get it" games, but be sure they are fun and not teasing. Don't pull the object away just when the baby reaches it. Let her or him enjoy success. The general rule is still responsiveness to the baby.

The daily grind goes on, and feeding becomes an even more important social event. Since you are varying the menu and since you may be placing your child in an infant seat instead of on your lap for solid foods, much can happen to frustrate both of you. Your baby can resist your efforts more skillfully by getting rigid, keeping the mouth closed, moving the head away, going limp—or, after you've succeeded in getting a spoonful in, by spitting it out immediately or upchucking later. None of this may happen or it may not occur for a few more months, but feeding can be a disaster.

What your baby is doing is coping with the changes you are requiring. Resistance at feeding time is a sign of growing up and being independent, but it is also a sign of not wanting to change a comfortable pattern. We do the same. We resist imposed change, though we may not use the infant's techniques. If these are the messages you are getting, then read them. Try a variety of food. Try a variety of positions. Don't be afraid that your baby will starve. Let the baby find a comfortable position and manage his or her own body as much as possible. So what if some of the food gets on the floor? That's far better than holding, restraining, scolding, and then witnessing the later loss of food anyhow. Work with your baby on the timing (schedule) of feeding. Let your baby help set the rate (tempo) of the feeding process. Watch for your baby's cries to signal that he or she has had enough to eat. Don't overfeed, stuff, or force.

It is still important to respond to your baby's cries. Early response in these three months usually leads to reduced crying in the next three months. However, your response may need to shift from comforting and feeding to stimulating and playing. This shift seems to come fairly early in this three-month period. By now you know when your baby is crying from hunger or pain—and either of these needs attention. If hunger or pain is not the problem, it may be that your baby needs your company. The active child will seek you more; if your baby is inactive, don't wait for cries. Initiate. Remember, if your baby is quiet, you should start the action.

Feelings. Your baby will also express strong feelings—anger as well as delight. If the parent responds to the baby's anger with anger and punishment, the emotions just build up and may explode in destructive ways. Even if the anger doesn't lead to physical violence, it doesn't help either the baby or the parent. Your control of your feelings can't be taught in a book. But what you can learn is that expressing rage is the only way your baby can cope with either internal discomfort or too much frustration and pressure from the environment—which means mostly, you! Unlike your baby, you have some options.

First, recognize that the baby's resistance or rage is a message to you.

Second, take a look at what you are doing. Are you setting off the baby's rage by your handling?

Third, what can you do differently? (Let the feeding go; wait a while to do something; stay and play another minute.)

Fourth, for immediate relief, can you use the holding ideas presented on pages 40-43. These may break the cycle, but you still have to see what set off the rage in the first place. What you shouldn't do is act like a four-month-old! Sometimes that's not so easy.

Feelings are a very important part of life, and allowing your infant to express them is a necessary step in learning appropriate ways to use them. These come with time and future learning. Your baby will learn mostly by watching and hearing the way you and your partner handle your own feelings.

Generally, your baby will be far more positive than negative in his or her approach to you and to experience. There may be times of stress, but the pleasant times are far more numerous. If you've developed a relaxed, responsive attitude, your baby will be entering the second half of the first year with a solid basis for trust and mastery. The next three months build on this foundation.

FROM SIX TO NINE MONTHS

Each three-month period has some special qualities. The months from six to nine have two major milestones. The first is the rapid growth in ability to move around. The ability to explore, just entered at the end of the previous period, grows rapidly as the child becomes more and more able to control legs, arms, trunk, and hand muscles. The second milestone is an intellectual one. The development of thought and language becomes more apparent, although the baby is still at a very early stage. These two milestones increase the power to learn, to communicate, to maintain interesting activities.

Some children will first enter the age of exploration in this three-month period; others will have begun a month or so before. The individual's rate of development allows for a wide range of "normal" growth. Often, people seem to think of babies' progress only in terms of how fast they grow. Parents sometimes compare the age of arrival at "ma-ma" or "da-da," or creeping, standing, first tooth, and the like as though children were in some kind of race with each other. We tend to think that faster is better. Yet there seems to be little connection between the speed of arrival at some of the infant motor milestones and later intellectual or academic performance or personality. That is, how soon a baby rolls over or creeps does not relate to later IQ scores, unless the baby is way behind what one might expect. What seems to be important is how these motor skills are used to explore and learn. Timing is not all. The special combination of all the aspects of your child's individuality, supported by what you do, seems far more important than the rate.

The whole range of individual differences—in rhythm, mood, responsivenss, and activity rate—that was present at or shortly after birth is still operating. These differences will influence not only how your baby handles the increased motor and thought capabilities, but also how you and the baby together provide for and respond to her or his growth.

This may also be a time when the mother is deciding whether to enter or return to the world of work—another type of milestone. You will need to face and work out a number of questions so that your baby's development is not negatively affected. Part of this chapter will deal with this difficult issue.

SIGNS OF DEVELOPMENT

Motor development. Studies of the ages at which babies arrive at those easily-seen markers of motor development—sitting with help, sitting alone, crawling, creeping, standing with help, standing alone—show the wide range of individual differences among children. Some babies turn from their backs to their tummies as early as twenty weeks, while others don't reach this point until they are thirty-six weeks old. That's about a four-month spread! That spread seems to apply to all these motor developments during this period. So when books say "the average child," and your child is within a month or so on either end, ahead or behind, don't get either elated or panicky. If your baby was premature or had a low birth weight (below five and one-half pounds), chances are that he or she will be likely to be somewhat older when reaching these points. If diet is good and you have allowed arms and legs unrestricted movement in the crib, you needn't try to "push" development—nor would any such effort be fruitful.

Given this precaution, you can reasonably expect that your baby will arrive at sitting by himself or herself sometime about twenty-eight weeks, and will follow this, in a few weeks, with creeping and crawling (getting more "open space" between the baby and the floor). Some babies creep before they crawl, and others do the reverse. About a week or so later, your baby will start to stand with help.

Each of these skills is not arrived at suddenly. Several weeks of practice and trial and error will precede each development—which is why your baby needs a place and time for unrestricted movement. The first attempts are clumsy, but the body, with practice, gets more and more coordinated, making the baby's movements smoother and faster.

These large-muscle (trunk, arm, leg) developments considerably increase your baby's range of action. Small-muscle (hand and finger) development also takes place in these three months. Your baby will be able to move his or her thumb toward the palm about the middle of this time span and, toward the end of it (before nine months), may be able to touch the end of the thumb to the tip of a finger. Think what that means: by nine months your baby can move toward an object under his or her own motor power, pick it up with precision, hold and examine it. The opposed thumb is one of the great, special qualities of humans—it enables us to use tools, turn dials, write. But it also enables babies to pull plugs out of electric sockets, open cupboard drawers, and get into other unsafe situations. Like everything else about growing up and being human, it is a mixed blessing, depending on what the baby does with the ability and how you respond to what he or she does.

Intellectual development.

The baby's mind, of course, is not easily read. Psychologists guess what's going on from what they see. They put themselves, to some degree, inside the child's mind. One thing is clear: babies don't think like adults, but have a logic all their own. We can guess this from watching what they do in certain situations. We obviously can't ask them why they do it, but we can make pretty good guesses when many babies do the same types of things in similar circumstances.

You can do this, too, to get an idea of your baby's thoughts. You can see the difference between how you think and how your baby thinks by his or her responses to your comings and goings, and to the removal or disappearance of toys or objects. You know that just because you can't see another person or an object, this doesn't mean the person or object doesn't exist. But for the very young infant, it appears, out of sight is out of mind.

62

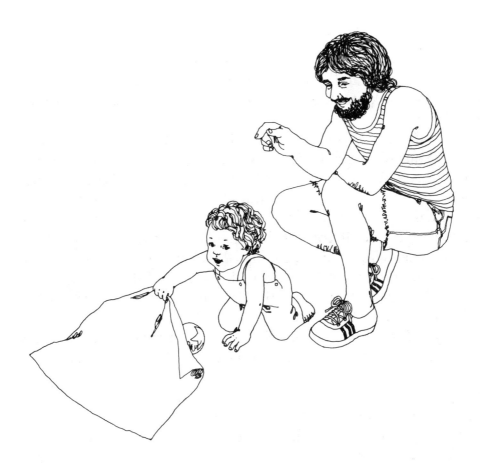

It takes quite a bit of time, beginning around the age of six months, for the child to discover that people and objects exist even when they can't be seen. Since you, the parent, are such an important object—if you don't mind being called that—to your baby, you achieve some permanence in his or her mind about this time. Your baby, when looking at you, listening to you, being held by you, has known for a while that you look, sound, and feel different from others. But now your baby will show you that he or she expects you to appear when called, or come back into sight when you've ducked out of the room for a moment. The baby's eyes will be on the door, waiting for you to show up. Before this time, when you left, the baby lost interest in you and concentrated on whatever was visible.

You can notice the beginnings of "search" behavior if your baby is playing with an object and drops it. About this age she or he will try to find it. Before this time it was "out of sight, out of mind." This awareness that objects exist even when unseen is called "object permanence." It is a giant step forward intellectually; without it we could act only in relation to the immediate, visible world. All of science and most of human relations depend upon this ability. It means that you can think about the past and plan for the future. It gives you some security—you know the sun will rise tomorrow even if it is now nighttime.

To arrive at this marvelous point takes both time and experience. Your baby has to have experiences with regular routines, with objects, with people in order to attain the fullest development of this first stage of thought. Object permanence is not specifically "taught" by you through "lessons," but it can be learned well only if you set the stage and provide the variety of experiences with the world that will allow the baby to put various perceptions together. It is as though all of the first six or so months of loving and learning come together in the child's mind in one big discovery.

Baby Learning Through Baby Play contains some activities you can do both to provide experience and to see what your baby can do. When your baby has been looking for dropped objects for a few weeks, try this: Sit comfortably with your baby on the floor and let him or her handle an object, perhaps a squeaky ball. Have a soft blanket on hand, and gently encourage the baby to give you the ball. Place it under the blanket in such a way that your baby can see part of the ball, and with voice and pointing finger, encourage the child to find the ball. Your baby may look puzzled or may not search or may begin the search but become interested in the blanket and forget the ball. These all mean that she or he hasn't yet arrived at the idea of finding a partly hidden object. Make it play: show your baby where it is; *you* find it, with excitement in your voice—"Ah! There it is!"—and give it to the baby.

Gradually, she or he will enjoy the hunt and begin to look even when the ball is completely covered. Remember, it is a game, not a lesson. There is no grade to be given. Your baby is not passing or failing a test. This is one of a variety of experiences—and many may happen naturally during your baby's solitary play in the crib—that lead to the concept of object permanence.

Your baby will show you other signs of the growing ability to think. He or she will be able to use a tool purposely to accomplish some goal. Perhaps a toy that is visible but can't be reached is resting on a blanket that can be pulled. The baby, after trial and error in reaching, may discover that pulling the blanket brings the toy closer. Shortly afterwards, the baby will swiftly yank the blanket. He or she has learned about means to an end!

Like object permanence, tool-using shows that the child is putting ideas together. These are early signs of human intelligence.

Social development becomes another more easily seen pattern beginning at about six months. The social smile, which implies recognition of a person, is present. There are some special reactions to familiar and strange people. By the end of these three months, many babies show negative reactions to strangers. They don't wish strangers to approach too fast or hold them. Their faces will get sober, they may cling and cry to show their feelings. It's perfectly understandable. They are still working our person permanence. They've got the family members figured out—that they come and go but are dependable—but they don't know about others. They prefer a more orderly, reliable, secure world—and strangers *are* strange! If they've had many experiences with a variety of people, and if attachment is strong, they may not be afraid or anxious, but they are not altogether pleased to meet new people.

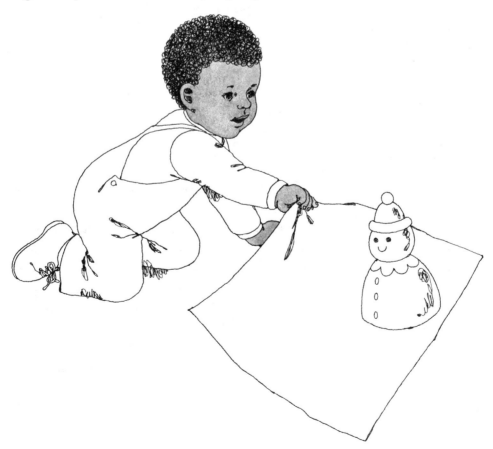

Just as they can intentionally work on solving a simple means-to-an-end problem, so can they intentionally copy and *imitate* parts of your behavior. Remember that even when they were a few days old, their bodies responded to the sound of the human voice. That was built-in, not really under the control of the infant's mind. Now, only six or so months later, the infant will spontaneously try to copy you. Your baby can't wave bye-bye yet; that will take a few more months. But there are plenty of chances for social play, for Ping-pong, in which the child's emerging efforts to imitate provide fun and experience.

These intellectual and social skills show self-development. Another indication of continuous learning about oneself is the child's response to seeing herself or himself in the mirror. Maybe this is the beginning of vanity about one's looks, but it is a delightful discovery for the child. It ties in with imitation, because your baby sees the mirror image doing the same things he or she is doing! Your baby will smile and reach out to touch, fascinated by the image. Don't bet that the baby really knows that the image is herself or himself and not another baby. That takes time.

If you have provided experiences and continue to do so, your baby will enjoy being with other babies. Social play can be seen among infants when they are in small groups and have had several chances to be together. They will look, stare, touch, and vocalize with each other.

Language too, grows in this period. Although not yet saying words, your baby can now respond to his or her own name—assuming you've used it!

An important social-language event occurs usually in the seven- to nine-month time: your baby will say "da-da" or "ma-ma" or both. This will depend partly on what you've stressed for your baby to imitate. Here your baby is copying your facial movements and sounds. The infant is putting several skills together, as well as refining physical development in the control of lips and tongue and breathing, to make the desired sounds. This has a powerful effect on the parent, and thus back on the baby. It ties you even closer together. Just as it was important for you to call the baby by name so that your infant would know and respond to it, you glow when your baby calls *you* by name! Of course, babies don't always discriminate very well. Even though your baby knows *you* are the special ones, she or he may call any female adult "ma-ma" and any male adult "da-da." It takes quite a while before your baby understands that only *you* are "da-da" or "ma-ma." But that doesn't take anything from the thrill of the first time!

Delayed reaction.   Your baby's recognition of his or her name, imitating your lip movements, showing intention, and the other advances in these months emerge because you've laid the groundwork in the preceding six months. There is often a gap of several months between the time you provide experiences, or the child has experiences through normal care, and the time the baby's behavior shows that he or she has learned from and is making use of what went on. This is an important idea. It means that your child is learning a great deal about words, sentences, even the rules of grammar, long before he or she can say even the first word. Through experiences and exposure to language *before* being able to speak, your baby learns that words direct actions, that things and people have names, and that words are put together in inform, ask, and order. Language development goes on in the mind of the baby when you can't tell that your baby is learning language. Learning, then, does not require any visible action by the baby that you have to reinforce by smiling or patting or nodding or repeating. It goes on in the child's mind as a result of being talked to and hearing adults talk with each other—by being surrounded by a language envelope. You are teaching your child about language all the time. If you become aware of this, you can be sure to provide the language opportunities that build communication ties between you and the child, provide models for imitation, and build language skill.

In the first six months, these opportunities occurred mostly during regular child-rearing activities. Now, with the baby's growth in motor and mental abilities as well as social awareness, you can provide, through social play, many more chances for language learning in a pleasant, informal way. Some ideas will be offered in the next section, "Things to Do."

Emotional development   now means that your baby will be more able to tell pleasant from angry tones. That's why, when you use your baby's name, you shouldn't use it just to scold. Your baby's feelings will still be expressed strongly, to show both anger and pleasure. Both body language and vocalizations show pleasure, recognition, and satisfaction. Your baby won't like to be confined and will engage in strong negative actions when this happens. That's especially likely to happen when you abruptly cut off exploration and free movement, and, for reasons known to you but not the child, place your baby in a confining space such as a strapped seat.

Individual differences also show up in the way babies handle fatigue, which seems to be more distressful at this age than in the earlier months. They will cry, whimper, scream for what seems like long periods of time. Active babies are more likely to show such distress. Babies handle their distress by the varieties of self-stimulation described in the last chapter: mouthing, handling their own bodies, and rocking and rolling.

Active babies are more likely than inactive babies to have more unpleasant contacts with parents. They are also more likely to get excited. This means that parents have to find ways to calm the active child through quiet social play rather than roughhousing. The inactive infant, who tends to stimulate himself or herself, may need more social excitement.

Sex differences get into the act here. Fathers tend to play with babies in rougher and more actively stimulating the explosive ways than mothers. Most babies enjoy this—they laugh, squeal, and chuckle—but such activities differ from Ping-pong. The parent is very much the actor, the baby the reactor. Babies may seek to continue such games. They'll bounce on the knee after you've stopped bouncing. But though it's fun, it may overexcite the active baby. You will need to match the amount and type of exciting activities to your baby's activity rate. Babies need a mix of experience. The particular mix has to match your baby.

THINGS TO DO

Environmental engineering. Your baby will want to move around more, and can reach and pull more things. Since he or she will also most likely be teething and may have a tooth or two, bite marks may start to appear on your furniture. Even the breast is not immune! Objects that previously went

into the mouth to experience now get used as pain relievers or as objects to be bitten. This means you have to check out the living space again. Survey what your baby can get at, then determine what needs protection. Each of the baby's new capabilities leads to the desire to practice. Through practice, competence is built. If there are books, papers, magazines on a low table, they will be Targets. Don't scold—move them.

Some people believe that the best way for a baby to learn the value of property is to leave things out for her or him to get, then punish the baby for handling them. While it is true that the child will eventually learn to leave those objects alone, she or he will also learn that exploration is dangerous, good books are to be avoided, parents can hurt you, and force is an effective way to control people. Are these really the lessons you want to teach a six- to nine-month-old? Control through fear and punishment has more negative than positive outcomes. Better to follow the ancient injunction "Lead us not into temptation. . . ."

Now that your baby can sit up, he or she enjoys the increased visibility this skill provides, but doesn't enjoy being confined. Think of ways to have your baby sit with the family at meals, with the least restriction of movement. This situation offers many chances for language exchange and observation of adult behavior.

Travel with the six- to nine-month-old raises new challenges to plan ahead. If you go by car, safe baby seats are available. Remember, the baby doesn't enjoy being unable to try out the new skills of creeping and crawling and trying to stand. Get a seat that leaves his or her arms free and allows a view through the window, without letting the baby impede your complete control of the car. Be sure to fasten some responsive toys to the baby seat for your baby's amusement.

Public transportation, especially air travel, during which one usually sits in a strapped seat for an hour or so, can be very hard on parent and baby—and fellow passengers. Follow the old Boy Scout motto: Be prepared. I've been amazed, over the years, to see how many parents don't know how to divert their children with simple toys, or games in which parent and child imitate each other. Instead, many parents scold and hold tightly, or they try to soothe. But most often, neither meets the baby's needs for activity—the use of large muscles or the child's emerging thought capabilities to play means-ends games and be

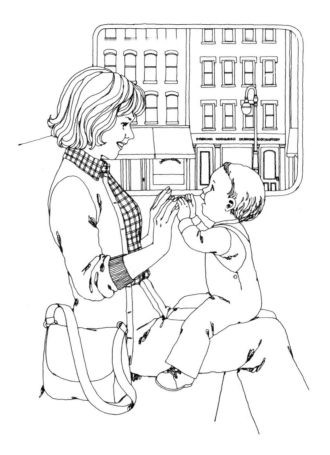

enthralled with "Now you see it—now you don't." As your baby gets close to nine months, you can even play "Which hand is it in?" by hiding some small object in one hand and encouraging your baby to open your hand and find it.

If you travel, pack an emergency ration kit of your baby's favorite reaction toys (squeak, move, make music); some toys for two, such as a piece of elastic that can be tied to a toy and turned into a push-pull arm-exercise game; a stock (in your head) of nursery rhymes that are repetitive and rhythmical. The words don't matter; the rhythm does. Choose some that require your baby to act, such as "Clap-Hands," "Pat-A-Cake," "This Little Piggy." Take along picture books so that your baby can sit and see the pictures while you make up a story and exclaim over the animals, people, or objects in the book. You may feel that this is noisy, but I assure you that your baby, you, and your fellow passengers will enjoy it far more than listening to you cope with a fretful, crying baby.

When the "Fasten Seat Belt" sign goes off, get up and take your baby, upright in your arms, for an aisle walk. Most passengers will smile at your infant without trying to touch him or her, and it can be a pleasant social interlude.

70

Remember, a baby who is fretful for reasons other than hunger or fatigue is usually seeking stimulation. Use yourself, toys and games, and other people to provide appropriate, interesting experiences for your infant.

Developing thought requires that your baby use the world around him or her. Your baby will enjoy developing and using the new skills for handling toys, people and self which reflect mental development. You can aid by the way you carry on everyday activities and engineer the environment.

For example, your baby will be able to stay with an interesting toy or object for several minutes at a time. This is especially likely to happen if the baby can control or manipulate the toy. You can allow perseverance to develop by practicing noninterference. If your baby is busily engaged in the crib or playpen—working hard, babbling, grasping, searching—leave him or her alone! It is a temptation to step in, to thrust yourself into the act, because your baby is such fun at this time. One reason the infant is so delightful is that he or she is working hard, practicing and developing mastery. Check in from a distance, but do *not* disturb! This applies in a variety of ways throughout the years. Children need uninterrupted time to mess and manipulate. Stay out of the action unless your child invites you into it.

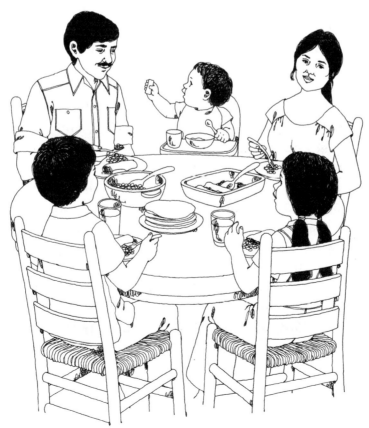

You can also help thought develop by using pauses and delays of short duration (three to five seconds) between your action, your child's response, and your next word or action. Mary Budd Rowe, a noted science educator, has dubbed this "wait time." It gives you and your baby a chance to get in tune with each other, so your response matches the baby's action. Wait time is closely connected to tempo. It gives you a way to observe and get your tempo to synchronize with the baby's.

Try it, even in a conversation with your partner. Wait before you talk. You may find your partner then keeps talking or breaks in on your pauses, so you may need to establish some ground rules. What the pause does is to break the immediate, "knee-jerk" response, and gives time for thought. It is an especially useful idea in language development in the next few months of your baby's life, but it is useful at all ages.

Since your baby is beginning to understand some simple connections between means and ends, you can pick up on tool-using. Your baby can hold a string or a thin stick of six inches or so. You can tie a toy to the other end and show your baby how to pull on the string to get the toy. Or you can use the stick to tap an object and make it move. Your baby has already experienced making the crib move by rocking, or getting a mobile to turn by pulling a string. These are what helped the infant get the idea of means and ends. It used to be "magic"— the child had no real idea of how his or her movement caused the crib to move or the mobile to turn—but now it is more conscious.

The baby is getting basic notions that *if* he or she does something, *then* something else will happen. Think of ways you can enlarge on *if-then*, and use words. When showing the baby the string-to-get-toy game, say, "If you pull the string, then the toy will come to you." That's better than "Pull it!" or "Get it!" The baby won't learn the vocabulary, but the explanatory approach rather than the ordering one does get through to the child. It shows up later, in the delayed-reaction pattern, when your child uses a reasoning rather than a peremptory language style. (See page 67.)

This is also a time to use and create "search" games such as those in *Baby Learning Through Baby Play*. Your baby will also enjoy other imitative and repetitious activities, such as putting blocks into a can and then emptying them.

Language play. You will find that your *language* activities will be getting more formal during this time. This book has already stressed that words should go with actions, so that the child builds an action list of words before actually using them. Words now can also let your baby know, through your tone of voice, that you are pleased, excited, or annoyed at behavior.

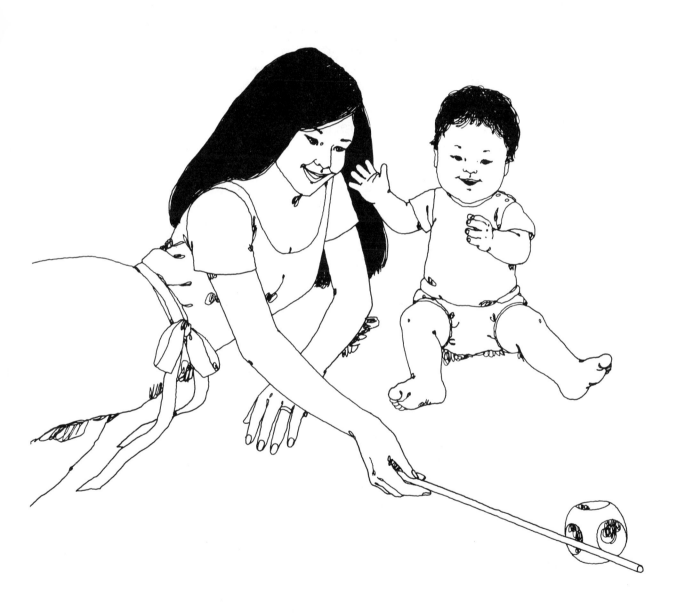

And you can label objects for the child, although it's most likely that the words he or she will use when words begin to flow (after eighteen months or so) will be names for objects that move or are responsive to him or her. By "responsive," I mean that your baby can do something other than look at or touch the object. Few babies say "diaper," but they do say "dog."

Through play and the daily routine you inform your baby that things have names and that words say what to do and express feelings. For example, an eight-month-old can easily follow where you are pointing as you say "Look at that!" Your baby understands, during feeding when you are pleased and say "Good!" with a lift to your voice. Words are learned through actions, not drill.

As a part of your engineering, watch the noise level in the home. Loud TV's, radios, stereos, and appliances act as deterrents to language and intellectual development. It is as though your baby learns to tune them—and whatever else is occurring—out. Babies "shut down" when too much is going on. More than that, these noises and words are not under the baby's control. He or she can't do anything about them. That's a lot different than the human, social exchange in which your baby's actions change your behavior, and yours changes his or hers. Hearing "Look at that!" from a TV soap opera is meaningless. Hearing and watching you, having you look at him or her and point to something to which he or she can turn and see—that's powerful stuff.

Make use of wait time, don't push for quick response, keep things light and playful.

Patience on your part continues to be critical. That's especially true when you feel your temper rising because your baby is not listening or responding to you or meeting your expectations. You may find yourself getting into a rising circle of demand-resistance-more forceful demand-more resistance, leading to an urge to punish and maybe even to actual physical punishment. You might even be thinking, "You asked for it!" But—stop a moment—who asked for it? Didn't you demand of your baby more than she or he could do? After the first resistance, did you take time to think, Why isn't my baby doing what I want? Or, Why can't my baby do it? How critical *was* your demand? Did it cut into the baby's own activity?

If you were out in public, did your baby's behavior make

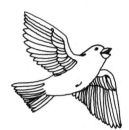
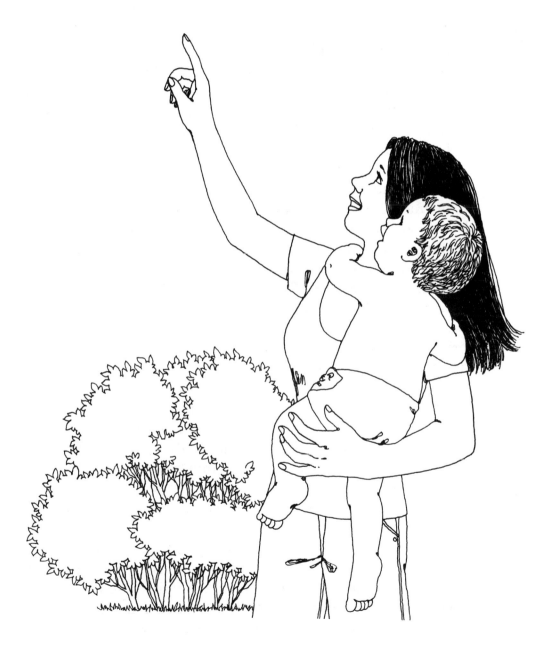

you feel embarrassed? (Did your baby cry, or—in a supermarket—reach for or knock over a can from a display, or point at a banana or some colorful box and whine for it?) Did your baby shy away from an adult friend of yours (who is a stranger to that baby)? Are you reacting to *your* feelings and forgetting that, in spite of the growth these last months, your baby is still an infant? Active babies especially will have unpleasant moments when they are out of harmony with you. Don't increase the level of friction; try to remember how little and vulnerable your infant really is.

Care outside the home.
Since your baby is still so young and vulnerable, and has, in these three months, become warier of strangers, what about care outside the home? Your baby has been out among strangers, but you have always been with him or her. A useful step is to join with other young parents in arranging informal get-togethers in different homes. Again, you are with your baby, but the baby can become more aware of and interact with other babies and their parents. This may gradually lead to some voluntary "time out" arrangements, by which your baby will stay a few hours with other babies and several adults in someone's home. But careful ground rules need to be worked out so that patterns of care familiar to your baby are not disrupted. The members of the group need to share their ways of caring so that the normal expectations your baby has developed are met. Such a "time out" plan won't affect the primary attachment the baby has with the family, and it may be a useful learning experience for both you and your baby.

But what about *day care?* This means many hours of care by a stranger in a strange place. It may be a necessity if you have to go to work. Care in your own home should be your first choice, but this may cost much more than placing your infant in a family day-care home or a group setting. There are *many* precautions you need to take before doing this.

The ideal care for the infant below the age of one is on a one-to-one basis. Your infant needs continuity of care by a loving person and the appropriate responses to match and stimulate development. Many day-care situations cannot provide this adult-child ratio. Even where there is a ratio close to one-to-one, there may not be sufficient continuity of care and stimulation.

If you are seeking a person to come into your home to care

76

for your baby, don't try to link this to domestic service. Care for your baby in your absence should be a full-time job, not an afterthought to house-cleaning. The Office of Child Development of the United States Department of Health, Education, and Welfare, in its manual *Day Care—Serving Infants*, edited by three experts, Dorothy Huntington, Sally Provence, and Ronald K. Parker, lists some characteristics of a good caretaker. This list (here adapted sparingly from the original) is useful not only for screening someone to come into your home, but for choosing a center, if you need to do that. The list is, in fact, designed for group settings, but you should use items 8 and 9 to acquaint the caretaker with your family standards and values, how you want the person to behave toward your baby, how you want the daily grind handled, and how you want the caretaker to respond to the baby's initiatives.

The good caretaker of babies and older children:

1) should be patient and warm. This warmth is the basic ingredient in the caretaker-baby relationship. Only with patience can the baby be helped to develop, and the caretaker weather the strains of this type of work.

2) should like babies, be able to give of herself or himself to them, and receive satisfaction from what they have to offer. Must be able to appreciate the baby as an individual, since this is vital to his or her growing self-acceptance. A caretaker also needs to have a sense of humor.

3) should understand that the baby needs more than simple physical care. Should have some knowledge of the practical care of babies and be willing and able to learn from other people.

4) must be able to adjust to various situations, understand feelings, and help the child to handle fear, sadness, and anger, as well as to experience love, joy, and satisfaction.

5) should be in good health. Since the child possesses abundant energy, the

caretaker must be energetic and imaginative in order to teach and discipline him or her.

6) must be aware of the importance of controlling undesirable behavior, but must not be excessively punitive or given to outbursts of anger.

7) needs to show initiative and resourcefulness and be able to adapt to meet the child's individual needs and preferences.

8) must be acquainted with, accept, and appreciate the child's culture, customs, and language if they are different from her or his own. Helping the child develop a sense of pride in his or her own uniqueness is vital.

9) must respect the child and his parents, regardless of their backgrounds or particular circumstances, thus helping the child learn to respect himself or herself. The caretaker's own self-respect will aid in imparting this quality to others.

10) should be able to work with other adults in order to provide a harmonious atmosphere.

11) should have a positive interest in learning, understand the importance and variety of learning needs in a young child, and be responsive to the child's attempts at learning in all spheres.

You need to *train* your caretaker. Don't assume the person will think or behave like you, hold your values, talk in your fashion. Studies of the ability of children to cope with foster care in emergencies indicate the importance of keeping the situation as familiar as possible. The routines, food, and space arrangements should be as usual.

There should be a gradual introduction of the caretaker into the home. At first you both should be there with the baby—in fact, you will have to be there if you are going to train the caretaker properly. And the baby will need time to get used to the new person.

The caretaker, in your absence, should make references to you and say that you will be coming home later. Since your baby knows "da-da" and "ma-ma," or whatever terms you use for yourselves, the caretaker should use them too and talk about you to the baby.

If you must use a place outside the home, first try for a neighborhood co-op, perhaps one emerging from the informal group.

If this is not possible, explore a family day-care home, licensed, preferably, where only a few children are in the care of one person in that person's home. Licensing will depend upon your state or local rules. In many situations, anybody, with no training or supervision, can operate a home. Be very careful. Seek out your local social service agency, public-health nurse, or your local community-coordinated child-care group for lists of approved places. (The 4C groups are organized nationwide by the Office of Child Development.)

Then check them out. In another Office of Child Development publication, *Family Day Care*, Carol Seefelt and Laura L. Dittmann present a long list of questions concerning the home, the day-care mother or father, others in the home, health, and safety. They also urge talking over views about care and how to know if your baby is happy. For care of babies and older children, they suggest:

> Before you make the final decision about placing your child in a family day-care home, be sure that you are at least satisfied that:
>
> 1) you and your child have visited the home at least once while other children are there;
> 2) you like the way the day-care mother works with the other children in the home and how she will work with yours;
> 3) your child will feel welcome in the home by the other children or anyone else living in the home;
> 4) the day-care mother has a good idea of

what she will do with the children
during the day, that she has routines
which include rest, meals, snacks, and
play planned for at regular times;
5) the house is safe and comfortable for
   children—that there are not too many
   "breakables" around or sharp edges
   and that there is good light;
6) there are enough exits for the children
   if an emergency arises and that the
   children are able to practice what they
   should do in an emergency;
7) there are no people in the home, or
   likely to visit it, whom you would not
   like around your children.

The next alternative is a larger center, organized for children of various ages, with many caretakers. The same rules and cautions apply. In addition, seek a center that is family-oriented and welcomes parent involvement in the operation.

If you take your baby out of your home, you need to take special care that there are familiar elements in the new setting. Spend time there with your baby. Take favorite toys. Work with the caretakers so that routines are as close to yours as possible. Be sure, even after your baby seems established, to go back and visit periodically; this is not only so that your baby can see you, but also so that you can see that the quality of care has not slackened.

In the evening, you will need to provide special one-to-one time for you and your baby. The amount of time is not critical if the day care has been what you want, but the quality of your time together *is* important. Your baby will need this special touch from you and your partner daily so that attachment and security will not be negatively affected. There is, in the long run, no substitute for the family as the best caretaking agency for an infant.

When your baby is older, and if you've been at home, you may find that you wish to combine out-of-home work with the continuing home- and child-care role. For some women this is important for psychological, if not economic, reasons. What is important is to have a choice, to be able to work out satisfactory combinations of roles. Some women clearly prefer to be at home, and this is *not* a secondary role, if freely chosen.

80

FROM NINE TO TWELVE MONTHS

The highlight of development in these three months is in the area of language and communication skills. A second milestone is motor development. Obviously, these are not brand-new baby activities; we've seen their origins and development from birth on. It is just that your baby now can do so much more with words and with his or her body.

SIGNS OF DEVELOPMENT

Language.   Your baby's language skills are still not in talking, but in listening and understanding. He or she comprehends that words have meanings. Your baby can follow simple directions, such as "Wave bye-bye," "Get the ball (or toy, or doll)," "Open wide" (while being fed), "Come to Mommy (or Daddy)" (while creeping or crawling). Your baby will also know "good girl" or "good boy" if you say it with enthusiasm when something has gone well.

Babies learn words from parents and other people, and they learn them through *action* with these people and with objects. Ping-pong and passion are the main pathways to language development. Words are learned because they are used by the family every day, in various ways. The baby doesn't learn that

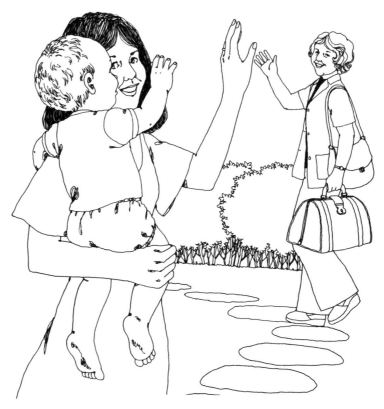

an object is called "doll" because you keep calling it that in a lesson-like drill. You don't sit down for ten minutes a day and say "This is a doll, now say 'doll.'" Of course not. You don't wait until your baby says "doll" and then give him or her a big smile and something to eat as a reward. Your baby learns the word "doll" from holding one, looking at one, being asked to hand it to you, dropping or throwing it, cuddling it—and by your calling it both "doll" and the doll's name each time you and baby are acting together with it.

That's why your baby will most likely, next year, speak about action-oriented or manipulatable objects or living things, rather than immobile things such as table, walls, floor, to which the infant has been exposed all along, but which can't be manipulated.

Action words become important in these months. Your baby will know "down" and "up"—and may, by one year, use them to signal you that he or she wants to be put down or picked up. It will be almost another year before most babies will put two words together—one an object and the other a verb—but your baby will understand your sentences now. This is another case of delayed reaction, that is, new evidence, in your child's behavior, of earlier months' experiences. Your baby's language is what is called "receptive." This means words in sentences are heard and understood, if simple and connected to visible things and acts.

Expressive language—the baby's own speech—follows several months behind this, in the second year and especially the third year of life. But the expressive won't be as full and rich as it could be if much action and exposure to *words in action* don't take place in this first year. Babies learn a great deal about people, life, and words before they can show what they know.

Since it is so easy to talk *at* baby, not to or with one, guard against lecturing instead of Ping-pong. The important idea the baby needs to get is that words have meanings. Your chattering away doesn't help him or her get that idea. Neither does TV or radio talk help. Your baby needs words *with* actions. These three months offer great chances for language development because of your child's increased ability to respond to your words.

Social development.
Your baby will be able and willing to follow simple verbal instructions, will show you things, offer objects to you, express simple wishes, and start the Ping-pong game. These increased social activities are all tied to increased language ability. They are the baby's acts, but they come about partly because you modeled this behavior in the preceding three months. They are evidence that the baby has learned, has understood the ideas of social interaction, and can show initiative.

During research at the Institute for the Development of Human Resources, my colleagues and I found that, among the families with whom we worked, these months were the ones in which the amount of Ping-pong was the highest of the year. In addition, the amount of Ping-pong we saw between thirty-seven and forty-nine weeks of age was related to the performance of babies, especially girls, on such activities at age one as knowing when to "pop" in "Pop Goes the Weasel." Why? Through Ping-pong with words and actions your baby is learning to expect a signal to do something. Your baby learns to anticipate that something is going to happen, gets set for it, and then enjoys the fulfillment of expectation. You'll see this later on when you are reading familiar stories aloud. You'll stop before finishing a sentence, and your child, with glee and without being told, will finish it for you.

This ability to pay attention and to anticipate a signal is not only a sign of thought; it also shows social awareness and a sense that things follow some order. These are very important ideas to learn, and your nine- to twelve-month-old is learning them through playing with you.

Development of thought is all wrapped up with

social and language growth. Now is the time when your child enjoys peekaboo and hide-and-seek. These are great games because they reinforce your child's developing idea that something you can't see may still be there (remember object permanence?), encourage social imitation of your actions, and use words as clues to act or to anticipate action by others. But remember, your baby is still a baby. Part of the fun is that your baby does not yet understand that when he or she covers the eyes and can't see you, you can still see him or her! That ability to put yourself in someone else's spot is still far in the future.

Games in which you and your baby take turns, such as handing or rolling a ball back and forth, now become fun. Social aspects and language are both parts of the game. If the ball gets to you, and you say "Thank you," it won't be long before your baby will be saying some short version, such as "Koo." Your baby may say this when handing you or offering you an object, and there will be the few months' lag time—the delayed reaction—before "thank you" in its short form ends the exchange instead of beginning it. But the idea is there.

Large- and small-muscle development and

use are continuing. It is an interesting area because your baby is now working on several goals at once. First, your infant is simply increasing his or her agility of movement. Creeping, crawling, standing, and then walking with help are fun for the baby simply to do for the sake of doing. Skill leads to use—which leads to more skill.

Then, a new element enters the picture. Your baby now puts agility to use to accomplish some other aim. Just as using a tool (blanket, string, stick) serves to bring an object close to hand, the agility of the body itself now becomes a tool. Your baby will creep or crawl to get to or away from some object or person. Your baby will use grasping skills to hold not just any object (as in the grasping reflex at birth), but to hold particular objects. So thought and planning get tied in with increased motor skill. This will become even more obvious between the ages two and five, when your child will creep as part of a "cowboys and Indians" or other hide-and-seek game, rock in a rocker, hold a doll while playing "parent," or engage in many other imaginative play activities.

If you have played a variety of hide-and-seek games (with toys hidden under blankets or in boxes) or provided many natural chances for your baby to discover that objects do exist when hidden, the baby, by the age of one, will almost always successfully search for an object when it has been hidden more than once under the same cover.

The baby will also enjoy putting small objects in a slotted container, filling and emptying cans or boxes. Although these activities may look dull and repetitive to you, your baby finds them intriguing. He or she also enjoys some block play, making two or three block towers and seeing them tumble—especially if you happen to be around to say "Ka-boom!" when a tower crashes.

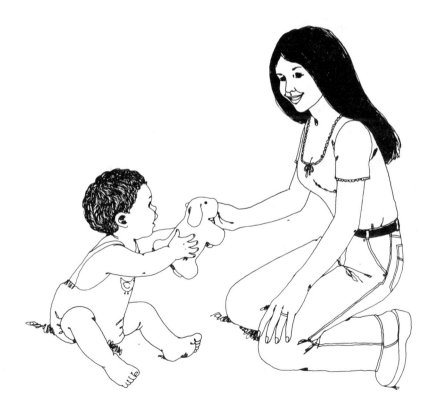

All these activities put hand and mind together. They also show the baby's increased ability to play by himself or herself. You can see *perseverance* at work. You need to be sure the setting is safe—small objects *can* be swallowed—but otherwise your baby can go it alone for quite a period of time.

The Daily Routine takes on new dimensions.

Feeding will become a new adventure as your baby does some finger feeding and shows more clearly both preferences and dislikes for certain foods. Since getting around—creeping, crawling, standing, walking—is so vital, and your baby will want to do these activities, feeding can be a time of disruption. Your baby may not want to sit still, and you may have to mildly restrain him or her in a high chair or other seat. When my wife and I took our babies out to dinner with us, we used for each two large cloth napkins tied together and wrapped around the baby's tummy and the back of the chair. This left hands and feet free to move, but provided both safety and sufficient stability so that the baby could eat with us. They were busy, active babies, at that!

Your baby may be torn between wanting to eat—and opening the mouth wide as the spoon approaches—and wanting to move, so that head and body turn away and the spoon hits the cheek. This can make you hit the roof! Fall back on environmental engineering: spread some protection on the floor for spills, keep a damp cloth handy for mopping-up and face-cleaning operations, and practice counting to ten. The pause may not refresh, but it helps.

Feelings of discomfort are a natural part of your baby's development. During these months your baby may show some fears—of strangers, of being left alone in the room, of the dark, of funny-looking objects. This is natural. Put yourself in your baby's place: you know your parents will pretty much come when you cry; you know what your parents look, feel, and smell like, and what their touch is like; you have some favorite playthings; and you've explored the familiar territory in your home and have been other places. You also have some ideas—though they are incomplete—about yourself. You know where your body ends and the world begins. You know that sometimes you hurt (as you do during teething), and you can't help yourself. You know that getting fed and changed and comforted

86

still depends upon people much bigger and stronger than you. You can do some things (such as creep) on your own, when these big, strong people let you, but you really depend on them. Is it any wonder you are afraid when they go away, or someone new comes at you?

Of course, some babies show little fear, others a great deal. We really don't know what is going on in the mind of the baby. We have a hard time knowing what's going on in our own minds! Adults have real fears, and we are anxious about things that others tell us are unreal. Why shouldn't your baby, too, show fear?

Your baby will get angry when he or she fails to achieve some goal, such as reaching a toy, especially if the baby feels that he or she should be able to do it. This is why teasing is so destructive. It is *not* a game to the baby if you put an object just out of reach, and, just as your baby gets there, you move it farther away. Failure doesn't bother your baby if the activity is beyond him or her. If your baby can't follow the rules of peekaboo, he or she won't be upset. It's *your* game—and your rules—not the baby's! But when your baby can do something and knows it, and you thwart or prevent action by teasing or confining the baby, then watch out!

Delightful expressions of *affection and love* also become more openly shown in these months. Your baby will hug you, will ask to be carried, will cuddle and kiss. Imitation, smiling, and seeking social play will all be signs that the baby enjoys being with you.

Your baby will be curious and interested in new toys. Although new people may be scary, new toys are attractive. By the time your baby is a year old, he or she will generally enjoy novelty and will prefer a new toy to a familiar one. But the familiar is still important, especially if it's a cuddly toy or doll that can be carried, dragged, and slept with. There are both comfort in the familiar and attraction to the new.

To sum up.
What you see in this nine- to twelve-month-time is how the baby, having acquired and practiced new skills of movement, language, and social behavior, puts them all together. This is what the distinguished educator John Dewey meant when he talked about "the whole child."

Your infant has come a long way in this first year of life.

The child is aware of the world around him or her, can establish relationships, can put some ideas of means and ends together, understands some language, can consciously (with planning) use the body to do things, can get around on his or her own power, can express a range of feelings, can identify people. That's a lot of accomplishments.

Some parents push their baby for competence. They may even judge the baby by some list of infant accomplishments, as though the baby were not a person, but a piece of equipment. Other parents feel a sense of loss as the baby develops. They liked the helpless child, totally dependent on them. It is as though their baby were a doll or plaything, to be handled and manipulated.

But the baby, from birth on, is a person in his or her own right. You can see each phase of development, each sign of growth, each indication of individuality as offering you an intellectual and personal opportunity to enjoy, cherish, and aid your infant. All ages are "good," because babies are intriguing in each phase of development.

Indeed, as a father of young adults, I can promise you that the loving and learning goes on and on! It is a lifetime opportunity for all—parents and their children—to grow. The details change with age, just as your responses and provisions for infant experience change during this first year, but the underlying theme remains.

THINGS TO DO

Environmental engineering

Safety. Since your baby is now active, mobile, curious, and exploring, you have some new functions as stage director. The first consideration is *safety.* Use the rule that if a baby *can* get in trouble, *your* baby *will.* Don't go overboard and so shelter your infant that you deny her or him experience. But check around and prepare. Make a list of possible dangers, and see yourself as an environmental protection agency. In this case, you are protecting both your baby and the environment—and your own peace of mind.

What to do?

Cover *all* unused electric outlets with a plug cover.

Cut all cord loops (drapes, Venetian blinds) to prevent strangulation.

Remove all loose and long wires.

Lock up all medicines, pills, cleaning liquids and supplies, sprays—all "swallowables."

Rearrange furniture so that the baby's pulling himself or herself up to standing, and eventual climbing cannot create danger. If your small, low stools or ottomans have coasters, remove them so that they won't roll out from under the baby as he or she uses them for standing practice.

If your baby has access to a yard or street, fence it or barricade it in some way. Do this long before your baby can walk by himself or herself, so that the child gets used to a large space with clear physical limits.

Don't have the type of fence or gate in which your baby's head, limbs, fingers, or toes can get caught.

If you have stairs or other "off-limits" areas, gates are useful.

Use a night light in the baby's room. If there's a bump or a cry in the night, you can check fast. The light may also be a comfort to the baby.

Another aspect of safety engineering is preparation for emergencies. Keep a good first-aid list handy. Buy and know how to use a good thermometer. List, in a prominent place, key phone numbers: doctors, ambulance service, police, fire, poison control center. If you work and your baby is home with a caretaker, be sure the caretaker knows how to reach you at any time.

When selecting bedding and clothing, check on fire resistance and any dangerous fumes that the materials might create. Be sure to also check if the materials may have any side effects. One safety precaution for the use of fire-resistant sleepclothes is to wash them several times before use. You might also check a good consumer magazine, or your local consumer protection agency for the latest information. Your local fire department will be glad to check your house for possible trouble spots.

Convenience is another good reason for a planned environment. Earlier I mentioned the feeding situation. Try a plastic drop-cloth on the floor. It'll save both aggravation and cleaning time. Cover furniture with easy-to-launder materials so you don't have to get into the "NO!" habit.

Opportunities for exploration and learning also can be engineered. Equip the play area, or whatever space gets used for solitary play, with blocks, empty tin cans (be sure the edges are smooth), pots, pans, small cartons, shoe boxes, dolls, and whatever else your baby enjoys. You may find that one use your baby makes of some of these items is to turn them into hats! Try to mix old and new, and avoid clutter. Too many toys are distracting; too few are sterile. Watch your baby at play, from a distance, and then judge for yourself what is a reasonable number.

Your baby will spend almost half a waking day in looking at and playing with objects, so you want to be sure that they are interesting, responsive to handling, and safe. Cans, for example, can be banged, rolled, nested, stacked, used to hide things in, filled up, and emptied. Blocks can be chewed on, put together horizontally or in towers, dropped to make noise, and used in a variety of infant-invented ways. The qualities of good materials are sturdiness, safety, and multiple child-created uses. Color and gadgetry are not essential. Wood is better than plastic; simple designs are better than ornamental ones. What is important, since your baby *uses* the objects, is that they can take hard use.

The emphasis here is on learning by doing. What does that mean for TV and radio? What I said earlier still applies: forget them as devices offering your infant opportunities to learn. They probably are harmful, especially if on full blast and continuously. For your infant they are noise—noise that detracts from learning and development. You may note toward the end of the year that your baby will watch and listen to TV with you. That's a trap; the infant needs other people, space, materials—not "the tube." I have stressed that language development rests on experiencing language in action—language used by people in connection with activities—and that your responses to your baby's efforts to communicate are vital. The TV can't respond,

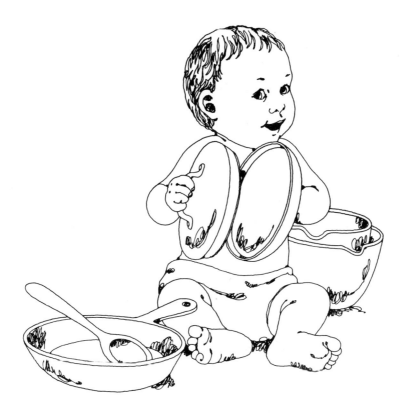

and the baby can't influence it. There are so many better ways for the infant to spend time, without the early development of TV-watching. After all, what can an infant learn from the soap operas?

Adult-and-baby activities.

If a parent is at home during the day with the baby, there are many chances for interaction. Most of the day parent and baby are each doing separate things, even though they are in the same room. Parenting is not smothering, and the quality of your relationship is more important than the quantity.

But there are three main times when you and your baby can be enjoying one another and sharing experiences.

First, of course, is daily caretaking. These occasions can and should be used for play. They can be used for affection—smiling, cuddling, stroking, grooming. They can be used for talk—describing, labeling, exclaiming. All these should be informal, unstrained, and natural; not planned, rehearsed, or structured. Lots of loving and learning go on in the normal caretaking routines; the touch should be light and easy.

A second time is playtime. This may occur at odd moments of the day and last for only a few minutes at a time. Usually, your baby will start it by coming to you, if free to roam, or by signaling you to come to her or him. This is the time for showing a way to do something, for Ping-pong, for getting on the floor and relaxing.

Here the ideas for activities in *Baby Learning Through Baby Play* can provide you with cues for what to do and how you might do it. But use your own imagination and creativity, too. There are many ways to play effectively with your baby. All include:

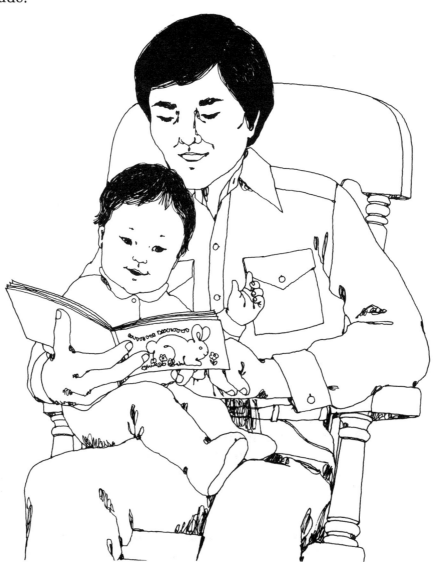

1) patterning like Ping-pong, with words, tone of voice, and gestures that focus the infant's attention on the activity;
2) providing the infant with information about what is going on and what is expected;
3) letting the infant know when he or she is playing well;
4) responding to changes in the game initiated by the infant;
5) keeping it fun;
6) not dragging it on when it is clear that the infant is ready for something else.

If you work and your baby is in a center or with a caretaker, it is essential that you have some playtime each day with your baby. It may, unfortunately, have to be planned, but it should be set aside. This is true in both two-parent and single-parent homes. The baby needs some high-quality, one-to-one fun time with the parents. You, too, need this. There is a poem by Longfellow that begins,

Between the dark and the daylight,
When the night is beginning to lower,
Comes a pause in the day's occupations,
That is known as the Children's Hour.

We've lost this, to some degree, to the cocktail hour. Think of how you can bring it back. You may find that playing with your baby is better than a martini—it is certainly healthier for all!

But a pleasure can be turned into a duty. That's *not* what the children's hour should be. There needs to be a certain amount of spontaneity to it, and what you do has to match your baby's needs, individuality, and state (alert or sleepy, playful or fussy, for example). One evening it may be roughhousing, another a toy-oriented activity, another just quiet time. Or it can be a mix of all three, tapering into quiet time.

Rituals become useful in these three months. You can set up some type of bedtime ritual. It may include holding your baby on your lap and going through a picture book, or telling a story, or singing some lullaby or rhythmic song.

Reading to a baby is an art form. It's easy to say, "Read to your baby." But what should you read, why should you read it, and how should you read? First, you are *not* teaching your infant to read. Don't get hung up with identification of letters, words, phonics. Reading to your infant should be for relaxation, and to create a later interest in the printed page, letting your child become aware that books and pictures are fun. Very simple picture books, especially those with animals in action, are good for beginning. Your baby has seen dogs, cats, birds, and you have probably pointed them out to her or him. Now you can show them in a picture book, and talk about them. You are trying to teach the child not that D-O-G is a dog, but that a *picture* of a dog can be called "dog." Your baby may not produce words that sound at all like the correct ones, but whatever sound he or she uses can be a sign of recognition.

When you read to your infant, be sure that he or she is comfortable on your lap, can turn the pages (don't worry about left-to-right—that will come), and is relaxed. Spend as much time on a page as your baby has the patience and interest to handle. You don't *have* to finish the book. It's *not* a lesson! When your baby begins to squirm, or falls asleep, or otherwise lets you know that enough is enough, take the cue. Stop. What you are after is for your baby to connect you and reading as a delightful experience. You are not teaching word recognition to the nine- to twelve-month-old; you are creating a pleasant mood and the memory that books are enjoyable.

Whatever you do together, you and your baby should be enjoying each other. You should show affection, and the ritual should enable your baby to go off to a pleasant, secure sleep.

Household routines. In addition to caretaking, and play/ritual time, there are times when you can interact with your baby while you are engaged in housework. The baby at this age will play by himself or herself, then come to you to "touch base." Your baby may need just a smile, a pat, a quick hug, and then be off again. This is part of attachment. Your baby has the desire to be in touch with you. Such times may just take a few seconds, but they are important moments.

This harks back to the first month and echoes the baby's needs for responsive adults. It's not a need that fades with time; it just gets satisfied differently. Look at yourself: how do you feel when people you love give chores or nonpersonal events (a TV program, for instance) priority over your own need to relate to them? Your baby, in her or his fashion, feels the same way.

94

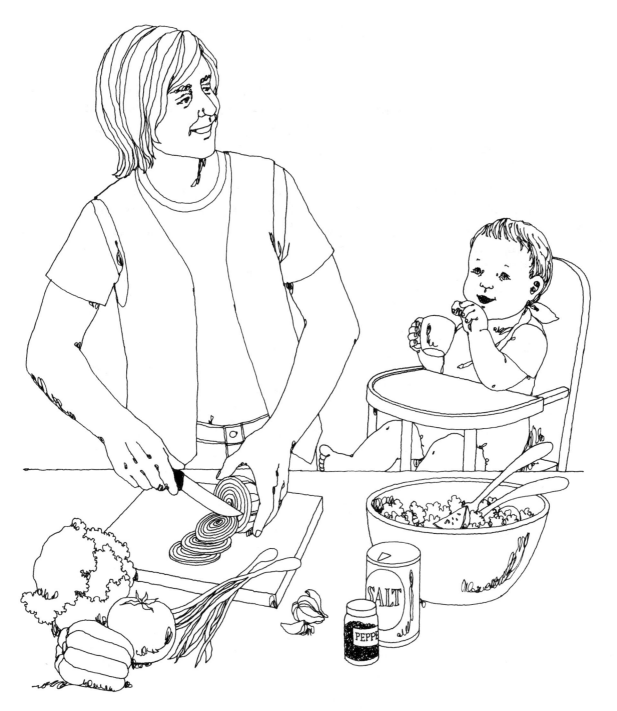

Think of it as the child's minute—and yours—a minute that will bolster and sustain your attachment to each other.

Of course, chores *have* to get done. But do they have to be done right now? You will not "spoil" your baby by responding to him or her first and letting the laundry, dishes, or dinner come second. Unless you are fixing a soufflé (and what parent with a mobile infant would be doing this?), whatever you are doing can wait!

Modeling is such a powerful form of learning! Your baby is learning about men and women from watching and copying what you and your partner do. You have seen imitation at work in sound and rhythm games, pat-a-cake, peekaboo, and in many untold ways. But here I'm dealing with delayed reaction.

Your infant, when more mobile several months from now, will want to do household chores with you. This comes from observing you at work now. In a two-parent family, partnership, sharing, and nonsexist role-taking become vital. Your baby, boy or girl, learns sex-role behavior from modeling what is seen. If both parents do a variety of home tasks, then the baby learns not only that these tasks have to get done and that the people who count do them, but also that one can be a man and do dishes, cook, and change diapers; and that one can be a woman and fix leaks, repair lamps, and bang in nails. The baby can also observe that everybody has to pull his or her weight to make the family go. Beginning in these months, the infant can "play" at helping; in the next few years, he or she will gradually get into the real thing, moving from self-help to helping the family. Although affluent homes may be fairly automated, there are still many jobs to do. There is an old cartoon, for example, in which Lady Bird Johnson is shown saying to the then President, "Lyndon, on the way to the State Department, take out the garbage!"

CONCLUSION

We began this book by offering the four P's—Ping-pong, passion, perseverance, and patience. Although your baby is now a year old, these Four P's should not be retired. They are useful throughout the child's development. As he or she grows, you will, on your own, think of various ways to use them.

They apply to relationships between the parents, too. The impact of the baby on the family's way of life is considerable. Even though you prepared for this and have developed patterns of life around the baby, the change has no doubt produced stress. During this year, you could handle it to some extent by focusing on your baby. But for the baby to develop well, the parents need to continue to build their own relationship. They need to continue to grow, to share, to be in touch with each other. The baby needs a children's hour; the parents need a "two-of-us" hour. This can and should be used for dreaming and planning. It can be a time when whoever was the main caretaker that day can describe the new and cute acts of the baby. It is a time for replenishment of spirit. It is a time for parental loving and learning. Take the time!

Since I've suggested you dream, you might dream, as most parents do, about your hopes for your baby. These can range from visions of his or her inauguration as President (rather a long shot) to hopes that the youngster will make it safely through the perils of adolescence.

Let me offer some dreams or goals for you. As I've talked with and worked with parents from many backgrounds in many places, and as I have tried to keep up with research, a set of goals has become clear in my mind. To match the Four P's, they are also alphabetized. They are Q, R, and S.

Q stands for a questioning mind.

R stands for *respect*—for self and others. It can also represent, on your part, responsiveness to the baby, which leads to the child's ability and desire, in turn, to respect self and others. The start you've given your baby, and the way you continue to provide loving and learning, should help your child be a self-starter. The goal is to enable the youngster to establish his or her own goals and to learn how to pursue them effectively. Respect for self includes not only feeling good about oneself and possessing a sense of dignity, but also showing initiative, drive, and direction.

Respect for others begins in the home. As the adults in the home show respect for each other and their child, the child will emulate this behavior.

Respect for others also requires that you provide your child with a variety of opportunities to be with people different from family members. This means people of a variety of ages, races, religions, classes, viewpoints, and values. If you are clear in your own views and present them to your child, then you need not worry too much that exposure weakens your influence. It may actually help, because as your child grows, you can talk openly about different lifestyles and about the reasons for your family's particular lifestyle. You'll face, sooner or later, the slogan "Everybody else is. . . ." You can reply, "But in our family we. . . !" Your child will learn that there are many ways to live, that he or she has a way, and that other ways are not necessarily inferior.

The S stands for one's own *sensibility*: competence, responsibility for one's own conduct, and commitment. People need to believe in their own powers, their own ability to make a difference in the world. This does not mean a false sense of perfection or omnipotence, but a realistic view of what one can do. The baby, as you've seen, comes into the world ready to make an impact, and begins, early on, to learn which actions produce results. That's the beginning of a sense of competence. You can continue to foster it by providing a wide range of experiences,

98

particularly those that show your child what effect he or she is having. The types of toys you choose, such as puzzles, for example, can show the child his or her own ability to solve problems. Your tone of voice, the rising, exultant lilt when something's gone well, is another way your baby learns to feel good about his or her achievements. It's best when the baby himself or herself gets a kick out of it, but your enjoyment helps.

None of us lives in the world alone. We all have responsibilities to others, and we need to learn that what we do affects others. You have certainly become more aware of that during this past year. At times you probably wished to be free of responsibility, to "do your own thing." You may have been able to work out ways to get time out—time you needed to get things back in perspective. But you know that what you do affects your baby.

Children, too, need to learn that there are consequences that follow their actions. Sometimes these are pleasant, but in the real world sometimes they are not. You can't and shouldn't shelter your child from the fact that behavior has its consequences. Experiences with other children provide a good way for this to be learned. When two babies struggle for the pail in the sandbox, they learn that neither is the center of the universe! Of course, safety takes priority, so if consequences are dangerous you need environmental engineering, to prevent them, or immediate action, moving the child swiftly out of danger, when they are imminent.

In terms of commitment, your child needs to know now only that what he or she does affects others, but also that he or she has responsibility for others. In the largest sense, we are all our brothers' keepers. Developing this sensibility, too, begins early in the home. Self-gratification is *not* the goal. Your baby is, and will be for several years, self-centered. But the idea of doing for others can begin with putting toys away, unloading groceries, helping with house-cleaning, setting the table, washing the disher, and, yes, taking out the garbage. Your child, seeing you do these chores, will want to do then *with* you. The key word is *with*. It's no fun for the youngster to do them alone. It begins as a shared experience. The child learns that being a member of the family automatically brings love—and responsibility. Self-respect, as well as a sense of commitment, is learned through participation in the family's routines, discussions, plans, and dreams.

You've begun to help your baby move toward Q, R, and S all year. If this past year has been a rich and rewarding one for you and your partner, you've probably moved yourselves to a higher level of Q, R, and S.

Perhaps our ultimate goal for our children, and for ourselves, because we too are still learning and are still growing, lies in developing a dynamic combination of competence and a sense of competence; a solid sense of self-regard and regard for others; and the ability to live in harmony with ourselves, with others, and with nature.